STEP BY STEP
REFLEXOLOGY

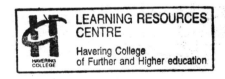
A simple step by step, easy to follow guide, which explains the principles and applications of Reflexology.

STEP BY STEP
REFLEXOLOGY

Published by

Douglas Barry Publications

Holborn Gate
1st Floor
330 High Holborn
London
WC1V 7QT
ENGLAND

Tel : 020 7872 5745
Fax : 020 7753 2824
E-mail: Info@DouglasBarry.com

FIRST PUBLISHED IN THE U.K. 1990

STEP BY STEP
REFLEXOLOGY
REVISED FIFTH EDITION 2003

COPYRIGHT 1990, 1998, 2003
© RENÉE TANNER

British Library – A CIP Catalogue Record for this book is available from the British Library

I.S.B.N.   0-9540176-4-1

ACKNOWLEDGEMENTS

My Family for their support, love and understanding given during long periods of confinement in my study whilst writing this book especially my husband who was a constant source of inspiration. My two grandsons Max and Luke and my Daughter-in-Law Sam who helped to keep me focused.

My PA and friend Jane Boland who worked long hours preparing my manuscript, interpreting my hand-written drafts and making sense of my thoughts.

My friends and former students Julie Quinn and Julia Wood for reading the final draft and making valuable suggestions.

Finally, both my sons who have spent their lives in a supporting role.

NOTE TO THE READER

This book is not intended as a substitute for professional medical advice. Neither the author nor publisher can accept any responsibility whatsoever for any health problem which results from the use of the methods described in this book.

The reader is urged to consult a general medical practitioner as to the cause or nature of a health problem of any sort.

MODERN PROBLEMS SOLVED BY ANCIENT SOLUTIONS

The therapeutic benefits of Reflexology, or manipulation of specific points on the foot, were known 4000 years ago, as this picture demonstrates.

The ancient picture is full of symbolic meanings. Egyptian physicians usually had professions other than medicine, with some being astrologers, architects, engineers, metaphysicians and scribes. In this picture we can see the pyramids, representing energy and the owl representing wisdom and learning. The three white birds depict health, peace and prosperity. The tools are representations of the instruments of trade, including surgical instruments of the time.

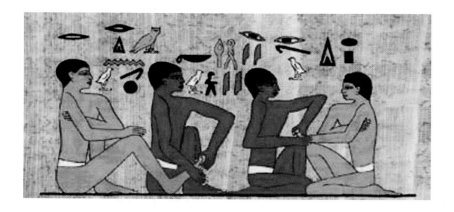

The inscription reads
'Don't hurt me'. The practitioners' reply 'I shall act so you praise me'

ABOUT THE AUTHOR

Renée Tanner is a world leader in the field of reflexology. She is an accomplished author who has made a number of appearances on television and radio and has contributed articles to numerous magazines and newspapers, as well as being principal of the first school of beauty and complementary therapy in the UK. Renée is an international teacher and therapist. Her clients/patients are from every walk of life, from every corner of the world. Many of these people make long plane journeys just to have Renée treat their feet. Her dedication to the profession is faultless.

A Childhood of Natural Health Interest
Renée grew up in Ireland, where folk medicine and folk-lore were a part of life there; where so many people influenced her in the ways of helping others, in particular her parents and grandmother. In the surrounding countryside there were those who had the cure for most ills: growing pains and old-age pains, chesty coughs and chilblains, to name but a few. There was the bone setter who was on hand to relieve the pain of a slipped disc and mend a broken leg, whether it was man or beast that was afflicted.

Observations and Changes
Following her nurse training in the early 1960's Renée moved to London where she began to study beauty therapy and later holistic massage and aromatherapy. Further training gained her a qualification in physical therapy.

While studying beauty therapy, Renée was fascinated by feet; the different shapes and sizes: flat ones, high arches, bunions (*hallux valgus*) claw toes and hammer toes, blisters and corns.

She marvelled at the wonder of these faithful supports that take us through life with minimum fuss, in spite of being the most neglected part of the body. Noticing that following a pedicure and foot massage most clients seemed less stressed than those who did not wish for, or have the time for a massage, she began discussing her observations with a colleague, Chinese therapist Candice Wong.

The Chinese Influence
Renée and Candice concluded that it was the massage that was the key to that special relaxed look. Candice offered to give Renée a special Chinese foot treatment; it was something she had learned from observing her grandfather, the local village foot doctor, at work.

Lunch time provided an opportunity for the girls to practice the therapy, but Renée's first experience of the Chinese treatment had her crying in pain, eventually insisting that Candice should stop the massage. Naturally others wanted to try, as Candice was convinced that Renée was acting like a baby, but each one in the group felt that the pain and pressure exerted by Candice was all too much for the delicate Western constitution. Candice agreed to modify her pressure and continued to work on fellow students during lunch breaks. Renée worked alongside, copying the act to perfection, eventually working alone and treating in excess of ten people a week in her spare time, including Candice, who had agreed to treatment providing that the pressure was hard and the therapy was known by the traditional name of Dr Wong's Foot Therapy. Eventually Candice gave the seal of approval; all others Renée treated about that time enjoyed the experience – with a little less pressure. *Dr. Wong's Therapy* was developing into a special routine, and Renée's beauty therapy teacher and school principal Marion Ayers was happy that Candice and Renée offer this newly acquired skill for the benefit of the clients.

A Foot Therapist

Marion allowed clients to book a treatment independent of pedicure. Chinese Foot Massage for Health was considered to be a more appealing name than *Dr Wong's Therapy* and so a new name for an ancient art was born.

This is when Renée first began to work out that there really was a connection between the feet and the internal workings of the body. At this time she intuitively walked through the feet in five or six rows from heel to toe, established today as 'zone walking' or 'channel clearing'. She also modified the general pressure increasing and decreasing according to the state of health, size of foot and client feedback, with regard to comfort.

A Western Reflexologist

Some years later as a qualified therapist and principal of the first School of Beauty and Complementary Therapy in the UK, Renée went on a trip to Africa, where she met reflexologist Edith Holmes, better known to her friends as Eddie. This was a chance meeting between two women at a social gathering and the start of a journey of further discovery for Renée. Eddie lent her two books written in 1938 by the grandmother of Reflexology, Eunice Ingham.

The First Beauty and Complementary Therapy School in the UK

Having given hundreds of treatments in Africa, under the supervision of Eddie, Renée returned to the UK where she added Reflexology to the school curriculum. On her return to London she also set out on a mission to find practising reflexologists in the UK and managed to locate just three therapists: Doreen Bailey, a disciple of Eunice Ingham; Gladys Evans, a disciple of Jo Reily, (Eunice Ingham's tutor) and, Joseph Corvo (a Zone Therapist). All four therapists met on more than one occasion exchanging ideas, knowledge and treatments. Doreen Bailey, who to this point was a therapist first and a self help trainer second, decided with some encouragement from Renée that she too should put her energies into educating and training professional therapists. Gladys Evans continued to work as a professional reflexology therapist until the mid 1970's. Joseph Corvo never deviated from his strong beliefs in Zone Therapy and continued to practice along these lines.

Pioneering Work

Renée realised the need for a broad knowledge of Anatomy, Physiology and Pathology for all professional therapists and introduced the first such independent study programme for reflexologists in 1974.

Renée was a founder member of the British Complementary Medicine Association (B.C.M.A.). She represented both Reflexology and Aromatherapy at the launch of the B.C.M.A. at the House of Lords in 1991. She later held the posts of Publicity Officer and also Education Officer of the Association. Renée has also served as a member of the advisory team to the All-Party Parliamentary Group on Complementary Therapy. She was a guest speaker at the House of Parliament in Cape Town for the Sub-Committee on Health and Complementary Therapy 1999 and was an invited guest of the All India Symposium on Health and Complementary Therapy in 1996. Renée spent seven years as Director of Reflexology Studies at London's second largest College of Further Education. She is the current Chair of the International Federation of Reflexologists (I.F.R.). Renée also holds the office of Honorary Principal of the Japan Reflexology Education Colleges and is an Honorary Member and advisor to the Korean Association of Reflexologists. Renée worked as a therapist and trainer in the South African townships and in Calcutta and Mumbai. In 2000 she wrote and published a document of guidelines and protocol on the practice of Reflexology for Cancer and Palliative Care. She has also contributed to the National Guidelines for the Use of Complementary Therapies in Supportive and Palliative Care published by the Prince of Wales's Foundation for Integrated Health in 2003.

Renée is currently an active member of the Reflexology Forum UK and of the Forum's Sub-Committee on Education and Training. She works in an advisory capacity for Reflexology in New Zealand, Australia, Canada, Barbados, the Philippines, the USA, Mauritius, Cyprus, Ireland and South Africa to name just a few.

Today Renée is respected by her peers as a leader in the field of Reflexology.

CONTENTS

FOREWORD

I first met Renée Tanner many years ago, when I enrolled on one of her Reflexology courses. One day, when I was arriving for my lessons, Renée announced to the group that her first book on Reflexology was ready for publication. That was the first edition and now, many years later, I have the pleasure of introducing you to the latest edition of this book.

Renée is one of the world's leading reflexologists and is a pioneer of the therapy as we know it in the UK. I have great respect for her detailed knowledge and her ceaseless enthusiasm for the subject. Renée is not just a teacher of reflexology, she actively treats clients and conducts research into the therapy. She is qualified in several other therapies and has written a number of books in these subjects. For many years Renée has acted on behalf of, or been a member of, some of the major pioneering bodies for complementary health and has worked to establish reflex zone massage as a therapy that is accepted by clinicians and hospital doctors alike.

This book is certain to become a classic text for anyone interested in reflex zone therapy. Renée's years of teaching experience are reflected in this simple, yet incredibly thorough account. The information is presented in a clear and straightforward manner, making it an accessible text for anyone who is interested in this fascinating art of healing. The content is relevant, discarding unnecessary information. Renée has indicated how to locate each specific reflex point and the text is illustrated simply by colour diagrams and photographs. Clear guidelines for treating a number of common conditions that may present themselves during practice are also provided. It is therefore a very practical and useful source or reference and would be excellent for those taking professional examinations in the field.

The simple and straightforward style is also very useful for the general public or anyone with little experience of reflexology. It can be used by those who wish to learn a simple technique to treat friends and family. This book provides the reader with a detailed and no nonsense account of reflex zone therapy and I am sure that you will enjoy reading it.

Dr Jarrod Hollis
November 2003

INTRODUCTION

Reflexology is an ancient art and method of healing which can be applied to modern ills.

It is both relaxing and effective. Reflexology is a therapy that requires human touch to bring about change to health and lifestyle and to encourage general well-being.

It is non-invasive in that it requires no pills, potions or lotions to be effective. It is also generally non-invasive of personal space, as the therapist sits at the distance of the feet. Reflexology treatment allows time to talk and time to be listened to.

Though not a panacea for all ills, it is beneficial for countless health problems. There is no age barrier to treatment. The infant can be treated as can the centenarian. Self-help reflexology can be done almost anywhere: in the car, on a bus, train or plane, especially if the treatment is given on the hand. There are quick and temporary pick-me-ups that will ease the stresses of modern living. Complaints such as headache or neck ache, for example, can be eased until a convenient place and time, when a more appropriate treatment can be found.

Reflexology does not offer a conventional medical diagnosis, neither does it offer an allopathic label for a condition, instead the professional therapist can make a reflexology assessment; a professional judgement that may be used to inform the client. If this is considered by both to be appropriate, this assessment could also be used to inform others, for example, in a health care team that there may be a need for further investigation. Reflexologists make no claim to cure, neither do they make a claim to diagnose, or to identify a disorder through treatment of the feet or hands, but instead the therapist claims to work with the body to encourage self healing. During a professional treatment the therapist will focus on reflexes that relate to the health of the client at the time of that treatment.

Contrary to some beliefs reflexology does not tickle, neither should it really hurt, but occasionally it may be a little uncomfortable on a sensitive reflex, until the therapist adjusts the pressure to meet the needs of the client.

Do you want to feel as though you are walking on air?
Then have a Reflexology treatment!

WHO CAN PRACTISE REFLEXOLOGY?

Almost anyone can practice the techniques of reflexology, especially those who wish to employ reflexology in self-help treatments. These treatments are generally carried out to aid relaxation, to bring about pain relief and to ease discomfort from many of today's common disorders (*see page82 Self-Help Routine*). That having been said, in order to become a professional clinical practitioner one needs to be prepared to undertake a long period of training. This is to gain a broad knowledge of anatomy and physiology (structure and function of the body) and of disorders and disease that cause effect and change, especially those more likely to be encountered by the reflexologist. This knowledge must be supported by an in-depth knowledge of reflexology and the underlying principals of linking the anatomy and physiology of the body with the specific reflexes. The student therapist further studies good communication skills in order to understand the needs, wants and expectations of the client. Other areas of study include nutrition and an understanding of the basic principles of other therapies, so appropriate advice and referrals can be given.

HISTORY, BEGINNINGS AND PROGRESS OF REFLEXOLOGY

The exact origin of reflexology in the ancient world is unclear. However, the following overview details the history as most well known therapists have characterised it.

China, Egypt, Europe, India, Japan, Native American Indians, and Russia - all of these peoples have stories to tell about foot and hand treatments.

America
With American Indians (Cherokee tribes) the tradition of treating the whole body by treating the feet in a specific way has been passed down through the generations and is still openly practised within the tribes.

Britain
In the 1800's Acupuncture was introduced into Britain and the first reported case of treatment was carried out in 1823 by a Dr Tweedale of Lyme Regis. In 1827 Acupuncture was used in the Royal Infirmary Edinburgh and St Thomas's Hospital, London.

English physiologist Marshall Hall in 1833 introduced reflex action when he demonstrated the difference between unconscious reflex actions, such as coughing sneezing and blinking etc., governed by the part of the brain known as the medulla oblongata, and conscious reflex actions governed by the spinal cord and decision making.

Sir Henry Head published in 1893 his discoveries about the correspondence between spinal segments, skin sensitivity and internal organs. The bladder, he wrote, can be excited into action by stimulating the soles of the feet. Charles Sherrington and Edgar Adrian explored the way the nervous system co-ordinates and dominates the body's functions and activities. Sherrington established that the brain and its nerves co-ordinated and controlled body functions through transmission of impulses. In 1906 Sherrington published his paper on the reflex action of the nervous system.

China
The ancient Chinese use many specific points on the feet to initiate healing. Chinese massage, as in Indian massage, pays particular attention to treating points on the feet. Local Chinese village doctors still perform a type of reflexology known as *Rwu-Shu*. Circa 2500 BC the beginnings of acupuncture in China are evident. Circa 1558 BC there is evidence that acupuncture in China had become more refined. In 420 AD a bronze statue was cast showing the location of all the acupuncture points.

Egypt

The Egyptians can trace their history of reflexology back to 2500 BC. According to an illustrated papyrus from that time, the medical practitioner of the day can be seen treating their patients' hands and feet. Circa 2330 BC (a wall hieroglyphic in the tomb of the physician Ankhmahor) is depicting a form of foot and hand treatment. The tomb was discovered in 1897.

Europe

In 1582 Dr Adamus and Dr Atatis published a book on zone therapy, through these writings we are aware of a form of reflex therapy being practised in the countries of Central Europe.

France

A neurologist Dr Joseph Francois Felix Babinski in 1892 discovered the Babinski plantar reflex. He discovered that by stroking the plantar (sole) of the foot from the heel to the little toe in any person over the age of eighteen months old the normal reaction would be the downward bunching of all toes. When there is a reverse response of upward action of the big toe, this is taken as a possible indication of a disorder in the brain or spinal cord.

In the early 1800's Acupuncture was practiced in France and believed to be brought to Central Europe by the then French Consul to China, Soulie de Morant, who became closely associated with Chinese philosophy.

Greece

Greeks do not seem to have written evidence of specific foot treatments, though we are aware of a strong history of massage. A number of medical documents are believed to have been destroyed in the fires of Alexandria. The Greeks made gymnastics and the regular use of massage part of their physical fitness rituals. Homer, the Greek poet who wrote Iliad and the Odyssey in the 9th Century B.C spoke of the use of nutritious foods and exercise and massage for war heroes to promote healing and relaxation. Hippocrates once said 'Hard rubbing binds, much rubbing causes parts to waste and moderate rubbing makes them grow'. Hippocrates's advice still serves as a valuable guideline for modern therapists. Hippocrates believed that all physicians should be trained in massage as a method of healing.

India

The peoples of India performed a form of pressure technique on the feet as part of their system of Ayurvedic medicine. These traditions live on through oral exchange and skills demonstration from generation to generation. The feet are thought to symbolise the unity of the universe and the ultimate one. An ancient foot chart contains Sanskrit symbols and although the true significance of these symbols has been lost over time, they do appear to have some relationship to modern reflexology charts.

Italy
During the 1800's Fillipo Pacini, an anatomist, discovered Pacinian corpuscles in the skin, joints and tendons. These sensory receptors are sensitive to changes of pressure. Angelo Ruffini discovered Ruffini corpuscles which respond to heat.

Germany
Johann August Unzer a German physiologist was the first to use the word 'reflex' with reference to motor reactions (muscular movement stimulated by nerves). Dr Alfonse Cornelius is credited with the discovery of the fact that spending time treating a painful area contributed to the improvement of health and the elimination of pain. Cornelius established that all conditions reveal themselves as sensitive pressure points which indicate imbalances in the body, long before they manifest as the neurological problems of pain. Reflex massage was developed and the results of the treatment were then credited to the results of reflex actions. Karl Ludwig Merkel discovered Merkel's disc, tactile end-organs responding when the tissue is stretched. George Meissner discovered Meissner's corpuscles, found in the fingertips and lips. In the late 1800's Hermann Oppenheim a neurologist, found that when pressure is applied to the tibial crest there is a fanning of all toes and an extension of the big toe this is indicative of lesions within the pyramidal tract. German reflexologist Hanne Marquardt studied in the USA in the early 1970's

Japan
Circa 500 BC Acupuncture reached Japan. During the 1800s an ancient energy healing system based on Tibetan text grew in Japan from the teachings of Dr Mikao Usui. His teachings were based on the theory that universal life energy was channelled through the practioner, who in turn conveyed it through their fingers to those who needed it. Reiki is now a well established therapy world wide.

Russia
In the 1800's Vladimir Michailovich Bekhterev used experimental methods of reflexology with animals. In 1907 he formed the PsychoneUrological Institute, and later became director of the State Reflexological Institute in Leningrad for the study of the Brain.
Ludvig Puusepp, a neurosurgeon, discovered that by stroking the general outer area of the foot in a healthy person there is little or no response yet in individuals with upper motor neurone disease there is a slow abduction (moving/taking away from the centre) of the little toe in response to the stroking.

USA
Charles Gilbert Chaddock, a neurologist, discovered that reflex extension of the big toe was induced by percussion on the external malleolar region (outer ankle area) and this was indicative of pyramidal tract lesions. Medical doctors William Fitzgerald and Edwin Bowers are generally acknowledged as the forefathers of modern reflexology. Influenced by Fitzgerald's trips abroad and by the Cherokee tribes of his native New

England, Fitzgerald was head of the Ear, Nose and Throat Unit at St. Francis Hospital Hartford, Connecticut. He also worked at the London Hospital in the UK and did further studies and teaching in Vienna. Fitzgerald, as early as 1917, discovered that pressure on the hands and/or feet produced pain relief in distant parts of the body and the condition causing the pain was also relieved.

Bowen demonstrated how he could apply pressure to a point on the hand or foot which corresponded with an area on the face and then stick a pin in the face without causing intolerable pain, if indeed any pain. Fitzgerald went on to confirm that the parts of the body which had such reflex relationships lay within longitudinal zones or channels. He traced ten of these zone lines through the body and called his therapy 'Zone Therapy'. In a similar way to Sir Henry Head, Fitzgerald found that working within a zonal area affected everything along that zone and he published his findings in medical journals of the time. Most of his medical colleagues either ridiculed or ignored his ideas. One colleague, Dr Jo Shelby-Riley learned the technique from Fitzgerald and went on to write a number of books on the subject. He also taught the technique to his wife Elizabeth and to a young employee massage therapist, Eunice Ingham.

Encouraged by Dr Jo Shelby-Riley his wife Elizabeth and Eunice Ingham gradually lessened the emphasis on Zone Therapy, spending more time working on the feet on the pressure point theory. Between them they developed a routine for treatment which involved working only on the feet. Ingham perfected her own method. Elizabeth Riley practised a slightly different method, adding rotary pressure points and twists into her routine, however both women were still working on pressure points on the feet, just the method of delivery of the treatment differed. Elizabeth Riley remained working in her husband's practice, developing her treatment, while Eunice took the therapy to the non-medical public across the length and breadth of the USA.

Eunice pioneered the use of reflex pressure techniques on the feet and hands. Initially she called her therapy "Compression Massage" and finally settled on the name Reflexology. Eunice Ingham went on to publish two books: "Stories the Feet Can Tell" (1938) and "Stories the Feet Have Told" (1945).

Eunice often faced harassment from the medical profession. At the age of 80 years (1968) Eunice was charged and faced a possible court case in New York for practising medicine without a license. The charges against this frail elderly lady were dropped before the final court action. It is generally believed that her advancing years had a bearing on the charges being dropped. Eunice later retired completely from treating and teaching the public self-help reflexology. She died in 1974.

My own theories are based on a sound knowledge and understanding of Anatomy, Physiology and Pathology, supported by a life-time's experience investigating other cultures, other therapies and other beliefs. I do not teach the Ingham method of treatment in its purest form, though there are similarities. Like her I developed my own technique and routine, while practising on my eleven thousand case studies to date, in addition to observation and treatment of a further twelve thousand pairs of feet.

This book, Step By Step Reflexology (5th Edition) is the first of its kind ever published and is based on my routine. It completely documents a full treatment in simple to understand language, supported by diagrams and photographs. It is now sold in most countries of the world. A number of books which have followed my own carry information and text in imitation of this book, with no reference to its originality. This I do not challenge, but live in the hope that those who read and practice this method will gain the desired results.

My future wish is the continuation of postgraduate training and the integration of Reflexology into the Health Services of all countries worldwide, so all may benefit from this wonderful non-invasive therapy.

MODERN PRACTICE OF
AN ANCIENT WORLD-WIDE ART

Doreen Bailey
In 1966 Doreen Bailey returned to the UK to practice reflexology having gained her knowledge of the therapy from Eunice Ingham in the USA. With many years' experience working as a therapist, Doreen opened her training school in the late 1970s. Renée and Doreen exchanged treatments and theories and even made specific arrangements to meet in order to discuss unusual cases

Gladys Evans
Gladys Evans was a retired nurse who gained her knowledge from Elizabeth Shelby-Riley while she was working in the USA. She returned to work in London as a reflexologist from the early 1960s until her death in 1975. Renée kept in close contact with Gladys, from whom she learned a great deal about people's reactions to the therapy and the possible reasons for these.

Joseph Corvo
Joseph studied Zone Therapy while on a trip to Canada in the early 1960s. His tutor, Franz Henbach, was a direct disciple of Dr William Fitzgerald. Joseph never wavered from the Zone Therapy theory, believing it already had a scientific basis. Renée met with Joseph on a number of occasions in the late sixties and early seventies to discuss the differences and possible similarities of treatments and outcomes.

Renée Tanner
In the 1960s the Author developed her Chinese foot therapy. In the early 1970s she developed her reflexology practice and her teaching practice, setting up schools in the UK and Ireland, which later expanded throughout many countries worldwide.
Renée published her first reflexology chart in 1973, then her teaching notes as a monograph in 1981 and her first book on Reflexology - A Step by Step Guide in 1990. Other books have since followed.

The Author has been at the forefront in the development of reflexology training and standardisation in a number of countries and particularly in the UK.

Hanne Marquardt
Hanne, a German nurse, was first introduced to the subject of reflexology when she was given two books written by Eunice Ingham. She spent some nine years practicing the therapy before meeting with Eunice Ingham in 1969. When she returned to Germany she dedicated her time and efforts to teaching the subject, later taking her knowledge and teachings to many other countries in Europe. Hanne published her first book in Germany in 1975. It was translated and published in the UK in 1985.

Dwight Byers

The nephew of Eunice Ingham has spent a lifetime promoting her beliefs, techniques and ideas. He was invited to the UK in the late 1970s by reflexologist Tony Porter. Both men had met some years earlier in the USA. In London, Dwight ran teaching sessions and seminars for those wishing to become professional reflexologists.

****

Douglas Bell

Fellow of the Scottish Institute of Reflexology Douglas spearheaded the training of reflexology in Scotland and the North East of England, working in this area for over twenty years.

Michael Endacott

Spent a lifetime dedicated to the recognition of complementary therapies which has encompassed reflexology.

Ann Gillanders

Ann emerged during the mid-1970s as a therapist and went on to open her own training centre some years later, becoming well known in the field as a tutor and writer.

Nicola Hall

Nicola emerged in the late 1970s to take over and run the Doreen Bailey school. She has established herself as a well known tutor and writer.

John Hopson

Who for a number of years was the chair of the Reflexologists' Society has given generously of his time for over twenty years in an effort to find a common standard of training and recognition for reflexology.

Clive O'Hara

Clive has given generously of his time and expertise within the various groups involved in the UK for agreeing a curriculum and training structure, to standardise educational needs and qualifications and to bring the task to a successful conclusion.

Wally Sharps

Dedicated his career to the developement of standards within complementary therapies which has encompassed reflexology.

Mo Usher

Though no longer directly involved with the progress of reflexology, gave of her time and expertise at the inception of the idea for standardisation and registration of this therapy in the UK.

Other UK therapists and teachers who deserve mention for their contribution to the field of Reflexology and Complementary Therapies are:

Wendy Arnold, Louise Bowden, Denise Brown, Beryl Crane, Necia Simmons-Davies, Heather Fleet, Daphne Gardner, Elaine Gibson, Hazel Goodwin, Alison Gough, Aileen Harris, Dr Jarrod Hollis, Jenny Hope-Spencer, Jackie Lee, Claire McGrail, Patrick McMenemy, Sylvia Povey-Kennedy, Elaine Syrett, Denise Tiran, Helen Vintner, Marylynn Williams.

The following overseas therapists deserve mention for their efforts in making Reflexology what it is today, in the following countries:

Australia
In the mid-1980s, having worked as a therapist for a number of years, the late Vera Shephard set up one of the first schools of reflexology in Australia (the Verona School) and dedicated her life to the promotion of the therapy and the professional training of others to an internationally accepted standard. Many of today's teachers and therapists in Australia owe their beginnings to Vera. Others deserving a mention for their specialities are Susanne Enzer and Elsa Reid.

Barbados
Ann Lewis has designed a training and education programme for the inhabitants of this beautiful island so they may benefit from natural health care at its highest level.

Denmark
Denmark has been a pioneering country in the field of reflexology and research. Peter Lund Frandsen is probably the longest practising therapist in that country. An inspiration to fellow therapists and a fountain of knowledge for students

India
Dr S. K. Agarwal is president of the Indian Board of Alternative Therapies and someone with whom I have had the pleasure to meet and work with in the past. This organisation was established in 1991. Since its inception Dr Agarwal has dedicated his time to the promotion and integration of reflexology and other complementary therapies within science, research and medicine. The role of the organisation extends beyond the field of basic therapy training, into social and charitable work. He has helped to establish charitable clinics and camps throughout India which give aid to those affected by floods and fire as well as bringing medicine to the street dwellers

Ireland
Anthony Larkin for his persistence in the setting of standards and his documentation of history through the years with his wonderful collection of books. Maura Barry for her steadfast contributions and promotion of the therapy.

Japan

Kazuko Sasai. Kazuko's mission is to link medical science and reflexology through high standards of education, training and research and to bring the therapy to an accepted level of competency and recognition. Kazuko is principal of the first purpose-built reflexology school in Japan.

Nao Oba has a vision for acceptable levels of education and training in reflexology so that reflexology gains the credibility deserved by such a therapy.

Korea

Ki Cheol Ham's strong leanings towards continuing education and professional qualifications, coupled with his long experience in university training, has enabled him to establish a professional training programme in reflexology and he has facilitated recognition for graduates through the professional reflexology organisations. His many overseas fact-finding missions were his way of bringing best practice to his country, for the benefit of both the reflexologist and the client.

New Zealand

Alys Noys, a qualified nurse with a passion for reflexology, set up her school in the early 1990s. Spreading the word, she travelled the length and breadth of the country lecturing to the lay person, prospective students and the medical profession. Michelle Higham is another therapist who deserves a mention here, having trained in the U.K where she also acted as an external examiner. Michelle returned to her native country and with her skills she continued to work for the benefit of many in the role of professional practitioner, lecturer and independent examiner.

South Africa

Jean Hale gave generously of her time in bringing Reflexology to the notice of the government of that country and the resulting recognition of the therapy and registration of the professional practitioner. Others deserving of mention in this process are Sharon Durran, Liz Graham, Ing Dougan.

USA

Mildred Carter (a direct disciple of Dr Fitzgerald) whom I had the good fortune to have a treatment from which then expanded into an exchange of therapeutic ideas. Kevin and Barbara Kunz, whom I admire but due to mutually busy lifestyles have had the opportunity to meet only once.

There are many other therapists all over the world who deserve a mention for their efforts and dedication in making reflexology the popular therapy it has now become all around the world; however space does not permit inclusion of their names here.

WHAT IS REFLEXOLOGY?

Reflexology is a science that deals with the principle that there are reflex areas in the feet and hands that correspond to all glands, organs and structures of the body.

Reflexology is a specific pressure technique applied to the feet and hands where all the internal body structures and organs are mapped or mirrored in miniature.

It is a simple non-invasive treatment which helps the body to maintain a delicate balance between all the systems.

In Reflexology the feet and hands are seen as a perfect microcosm of the body with a somatic replication of all organs, glands and structures on to a reflex point. The word reflex/ology has five distinct meanings relevant to this subject –

1. **The definition of the word 'ology' is taken to mean 'the study of that branch of science.**
2. **A mirror image or reflection.**
3. **A reflex is when stimulation at one point brings about a response in another point or area.**
4. **To turn or be directed back.**
5. **An unconscious or involuntary response to stimuli.**

In Reflexology by using pressure or palpation on a reflex point on the foot or hand, imbalances in the body can be both detected and effectively treated through a system of zones or energy channels that link specific reflexes with specific organs or structures.

Reflexology is a natural, holistic non-invasive therapy. The practitioner uses only the techniques of human therapeutic touch and does not rely on any implements or gadgets to help bring about results.

Reflexology recognises that the points known as reflexes that correspond to the body's structures, glands, organs and systems are not visible or verifiable either in anatomy and physiology or as yet by any scientific means. However, the effectiveness of these relationships has been proven in practical empirical experience over many many years and thousands of therapists and recipients of Reflexology have observed and/or benefited from the effects.

What are Zones/Energy Channels?
Zones or Zone Therapy is a system of discovery or re-discovery that established with the application of pressure to zonal points on the body (including feet and hands) a reflex action occurs within the same zone. This theory was first published by

Dr Adamus and Dr Atatis in the Sixteenth Century. However, credit of its emergence as a therapy and fore-runner to Reflexology must go to Dr William Fitzgerald an ENT specialist who worked not only in the USA as a medical specialist but also in London, England and Vienna, Austria, under the guidance of the leading consultants and professors of the day.

What is Zone Therapy?
In 1917 Dr William Fitzgerald together with Dr Edwin Bowers published a book: The title read '*Zone Therapy or Relieving Pain at Home*'. In this book Fitzgerald wrote that he had accidentally discovered that pressure with a cotton-tipped probe on the muco-cutaneous margin of the nose gave an anaesthetic type effect, as though cocaine solution had been applied. He subsequently discovered many other areas including those on the hands and feet, which when pressed deadened sensation, brought about pain relief and also relief in the condition causing the pain. Dr Fitzgerald also noted that the parts of the body which had such a reflex relationship lay within certain longitudinal zones. He speculated that the human body could be divided into ten longitudinal zones or energy channels, ascending from the feet to the brain.

In the human body the ten invisible energy zones are located with five either side of the median line. The five zones on the right foot/hand represent the right side of the body. The five zones on the left foot/hand represent the left side of the body.

Five on each foot represents a simple numbering system with the big toe in Zone 1, second toe in Zone 2, third toe in Zone 3, fourth toe in Zone 4 and fifth toe (little toe) in Zone 5. (See diagram, page 26)

The fingers correspond to the toes with the thumb in Zone 1 and the little finger in Zone 5. An organ, gland or structure found in a specific zone will have its reflex point in the corresponding zone of the foot/hand.

Where two organs exist, for example two lungs, then they will be found one on each foot. Likewise where an organ crosses the midline in the body it will then be found on both feet/hands, for example, the spine, the bladder.

Besides the ten energy zones/channels already mentioned, further lines should be taken into consideration. These imaginary lateral lines traverse the foot/hand.

These lines help the reflexologist to make a map of the foot and the body. It is worth bearing in mind that the shape and size of the foot and hand though basically the same will differ slightly in each individual. Therefore if treatment is always started by first visualising these four imaginary lines on the feet then it is easy to work out the reflexes that are above or below these lines.

TEN LONGITUDINAL ZONES

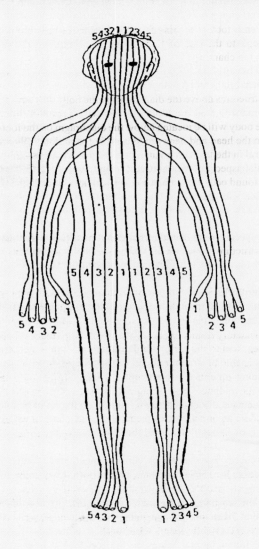

TEN LONGITUDINAL ZONES

Located five on each foot, stretching from the heel to the toes and through the hands from wrist through to the tips of fingers. Zones go through the body, dividing it longitudinally in ten channels.

Compartmentalising
All organs and structures above the diaphragm in the body will have their reflex point above the diaphragm line on the foot/hand and all organs and structures below the diaphragm in the body will be located below the diaphragm on the foot/hand. Reflexes corresponding to the head and neck are located in the region of the toes/fingers. The spine being central in the body, it is natural to locate the corresponding reflex passing through the medial aspect of both feet/hands (big toe/thumb side). The reflex zone to an organ can be found occupying the same vertical body zone in the feet/hands as the organ occupies in the body.

Reactions
A reaction on a specific reflex on the foot could be a signal that the corresponding gland, organ or structure might not be working to optimum capacity.

Important Note
The Renée Tanner Reflexology Treatment sequence described in this book is actually treating the whole body. Within the sequence routine, further treatment of the reflex is added, concentrating on the actual area of the reflex which has proven over time to give the most satisfactory results. Working in this way helps to prevent over-stimulating a particular reflex, hence avoiding or minimising the healing reaction (crisis). An example of this is the heart, which is treated in its entirety in the general chest sequence and backed up with further treatment of the left foot only, though in reality the heart crosses the midline. Another example is the liver, treated in its entirety in the upper abdomen sequence supported with specific treatment of Zone 3 to Zone 5 on the right foot. Working in this manner also helps to confirm reflex reactions, i.e. sensitivities, tensions, energy blockages relative to a specific reflex.

Eunice Ingham
It is interesting to note here that when Eunice Ingham, the grandmother of Reflexology, first began treating, she padded and taped some reflexes so as to cause further pressure over an area, which resulted in similar or more severe symptoms to the original presenting problem. From this she concluded that less can sometimes equal more. In other words DO NOT OVERTREAT REFLEXES.

Reflexology is not a 'cure all' to the exclusion of other therapies and to insist on it being so, indicates a lack of ability to evaluate the relative worth of other therapies.

LOCATION GUIDELINES TO AID COMPARTMENTALISATION

1. Shoulder Line

Located as an imaginary horizontal line across the sole of the foot where the bones of the foot (metatarsals) and those of the toes (phalanges) meet (metatarsal/phalangeal joint). On the ball of the foot, just below the ridge at the base of the toes.

2. Diaphragm Line

Located as an imaginary horizontal line across the sole of the foot, just under the ball (distal to the toes).

3. Waist Line

Located as an imaginary horizontal line across the middle of the foot, stretching from the metatarsal tuberosity on the lateral edge of the foot to the arch on the medial edge.

4. Pelvic Floor Line

Located as an imaginary horizontal line across the sole of the foot where the soft flesh meets the thicker heel pad.

5. Longitudinal Tendon Guideline (flexor hallucis longis)

Located on the sole of the foot between the diaphragm and the pelvic floor line it becomes obvious when the toes are pushed back (away), especially the big toe.
Note: This fifth guide is not used by all therapists.

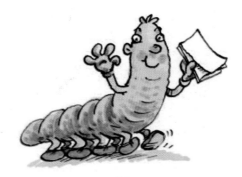

LOCATION GUIDELINES

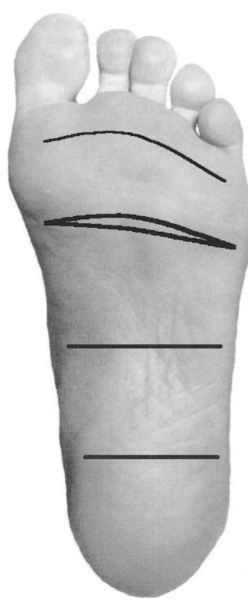

Shoulder line

Diaphragm line

Waist line

Pelvic floor line

REFERRAL ZONES

I have chosen to include this section; however the concept is still a puzzle to me. I feel we as therapists, have followed the idea through without sufficient investigation.

- Fingers Treat Toes

- Hand Treat Foot

- Wrist Treat Ankle

- Forearm Treat Calf

- Elbow Treat Knee

- Upper Arm Treat Thigh

- Shoulder Treat Hip

I can see no reason or time when a professional therapist might use these cross reflexes other than when working in a specialised area of disability. Even then the hands would be a more appropriate choice than legs and arms.

Reflexologists do not normally treat the arms and legs during treatment however in a self-help situation massage pressure or a zone walk on the cross reflex could in theory bring about some relief.

The professional therapist is taught during training that treatment on any reflex has an impact on all reflexes within that zone, hence, arm, hand; leg, foot, would be accommodated within zone 5.

REFERRAL ZONES

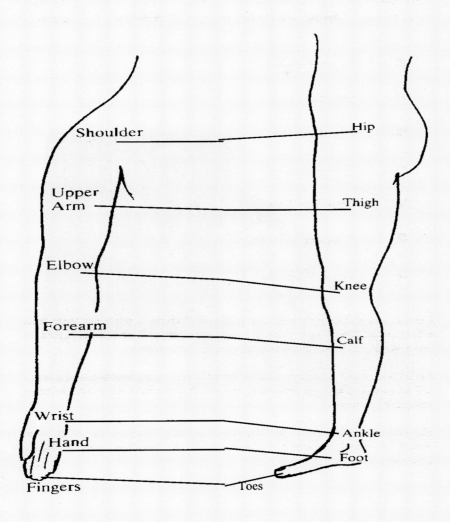

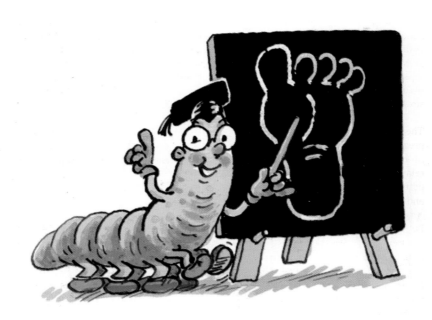

HOW DOES REFLEXOLOGY WORK?

As yet we have no definitive answer on how reflexology works. What we do have is a number of theoretical concepts on how it works. Making time for treatment is the first step in making time for self. Reflexology can aid in raising a client's self esteem and improve self image, encouraging the client to take a closer look at their health and lifestyle.

Sir Henry Head was responsible for discovering that through different parts of the nervous system, the skin can affect organs in the body and organs can affect the skin. He also noted areas of sensitivity lay at a distance from the affected part. Together with his colleague Sir James McKenzie they proved that therapeutic methods applied to the surface of a part of the body influenced pathological conditions associated with an organ or structure in a particular area. In proving the theory the skin was stimulated with various techniques of cold, electrotherapy, heat, manipulation, pressure and stroking.

The brain releases endorphins, which are the body's natural pain relievers. Reflexology pressure stimulates the brain to release more endorphins while at the same time producing an 'overload' for the nervous system, shutting down nerve pathways relaying pain signals to the brain. There are a number of areas on the body where large numbers of nerve cells are close to the skin's surface, these include the soles of the feet and the hands.

Dr Fitzgerald believed amongst other things that the control centres in the medulla of the brain stem are stimulated by the pressure and also may be influenced by the pituitary gland and nerve pathways from it.

Dr Jo Shelby-Riley believed 'Zone Therapy' worked by inhibiting pain through manipulation, touch and pressure before nerve impulses reached the brain. Eunice Ingham's theory suggests reflexology works by stimulation of the sympathetic and parasympathetic parts of the autonomic nervous system.

Positive-Negative Poles

Dr Randolph Stone developed polarity therapy, which is based on the Eastern philosophy of energy pathways. He believed reflexology works through these pathways. Dr Stone's theory involves negative and positive poles of electrically charged energy which stimulate reflex points releasing energy blocks, and restoring balance.

Acupuncture Theory

Some theories suggest reflexology is closely related to acupuncture meridians. Reflexologists believe, as with acupuncture, that when an energy channel or meridian is blocked the harmony of the body becomes imbalanced. Reflexologists work on both acupressure and acupuncture points during the course of treatment, but do not define the same meridian lines/channels.

Reiterative Theory

Dr Alan Dale, writer of 'Comparatives between Acupuncture and Reflexology' has suggested Reflexology and other systems which project the body whole on a part i.e. feet, hands, face are in fact based on Reiterative Theory.

Other Theories

Explain the reflexes as mirrored images of organs and structures with the location and relationship of reflexes largely following an anatomical patterning which reflects that of the body.

Some modern therapists believe results are based on the body's reflex relationships (physiological relationships).

The Energy Theory

Energy theorists believe that the free flow of natural energy is vital to health. Due to stress and tension, energy blockages can occur in the energy pathways resulting in disorders and disease. Reflexology aims to free the blockage returning the body to its normal state of health.

Placebo Effect

It is well documented through research that health problems have improved as a result of the placebo effect. If a large number of clients feel benefit from reflexology and a proportion of these believe that reflexology will help the presenting condition, there must be an element here that suggests reflexology works through the placebo effect.

Pain Gate Theory

Medical science has established the existence of reflex relationships mainly through the nervous system. A nerve signal is an electrical impulse produced by chemical reactions on the surface of the neuron body (nerve cell body). The reflex arch of nerve stimulation, is demonstrated for example, if you pick up a very hot dinner plate, the sensory nerves convey the information to the spinal nerves. The motor nerves initiate a response of withdrawing the hand from the plate. A similar reaction would occur to pressure or injury.

The Cellular Theory

Reflexology is unblocking at the cellular level removing toxic waste that has collected within the cells causing them to malfunction. Through neurological reaction this malfunction is eventually felt on the physical level.

The Foetal Position Theory

Reflexologists believe that the map of the body as mirrored onto the feet is based on the foetal position. Hence the knee is located higher than the hip (medial to the toes). I accept this concept, I also accept that when treating the foot the reflex of/to the hand is treated and visa versa.

Finally

Food for Thought

Perhaps reflexology could be likened to an electric light bulb. The switch is touched at a distance from the bulb yet when the switch is touched the bulb comes to life and fills the room with light.

HOLDING TECHNIQUES

The following is a guide on how to hold the foot while working. Holds may be varied according to suitability for the client and the therapist. However the therapist should be ever mindful of the dangers of pinching the skin while using a holding technique.

Why use Holding Techniques?
Seven main reasons have been identified to qualify the need for holding techniques:

1   To maintain client contact and transmit re-assurance.
2   To support the foot being treated.
3   To keep the foot stationary.
4   To avoid pinching and confusing assessment of the reflex/sensitive area.
5   To protect the foot from pressure to the opposite facet of the foot, to where the technique is directed.
6   To spread an area of the foot so the working thumb/finger can access deep reflex points.
7   To act as a platform off which the working hand/finger can lever.

Seven most commonly used holds with some suggestions for use:

1)   **Foot Wrap**
       Put the fingers of the supporting hand across the dorsum of the foot, close to the base of the toes. The edge of the foot should nestle in the webbing between the thumb and index finger; the thumb should rest across the ball of the foot. The hold is used mainly when working on the sole and can also be used for bending the foot outwards or inwards, or when pulling the sole onto the thumb.

2)   **Toe Bend**
       Put the fingers of the supporting hand, across the dorsum area of the toes, the edge of the foot will nestle in the webbing between the thumb and the index finger. The thumb will rest on one or more of the toes underneath. This hold can be used either when working on the individual toes, or when working underneath the toes, to bend the toes backwards.

3)   **Sole Support**
       Put the heel of the holding hand on the ball of the foot with the fingers relaxed over the top of the toes. This hold can be used for either pushing the foot away (using the heel of the hand) or pulling the foot towards you (using the fingers).

4) **Heel Grip**

Cup the heel in your palm and wrap your fingers around the Achilles tendon at the back of the heel. This movement can be used when treating the hip area, when treating down the spine, and when treating down the outside of the foot.

5) **Beak Hold**

Support the toes on the dorsum with the finger wrap. Use the thumb and the index finger in a light grip hold on the upper edge of the toe. Separate the toes so that a gap appears

a) Between two toes

b) Between the thumb and the index finger.

Starting with the big toe and toe two, move along the toes in this manner until all are treated. This movement can be used when treating the cranial nerves and sinuses.

6) **Fist Support**

Make a fist then use the back of your knuckles against the outer edge of the foot, on a level with the pelvic line. Keep your thumb loose ready to walk around the heel edge to the inside on level with the pelvic line.

7) **Finger and Thumb Grip**

Use the index finger and thumb to grip the toe on either side. Pull the toe towards you. The index finger of the working hand can then treat the dorsum of the toes/foot.

1)   **Foot Wrap**

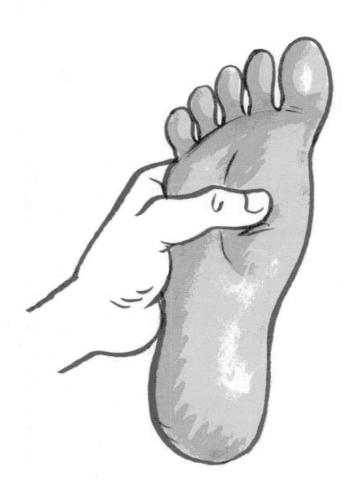

2)   Toe Bend

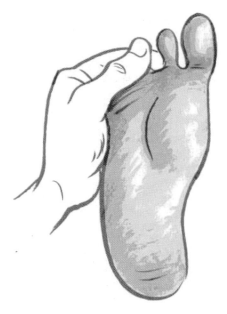

3)   Sole Support

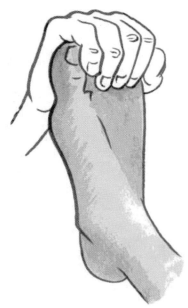

39

4)   **Heel Grip**

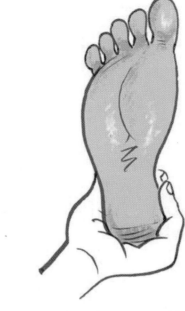

5)   **Beak Hold**

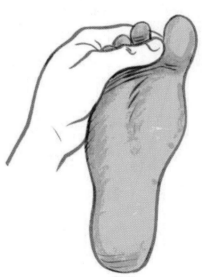

6)   **Fist Support**

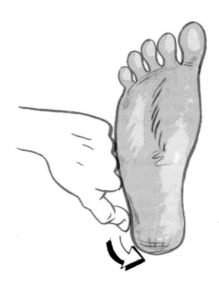

7)   **Finger and Thumb Grip**

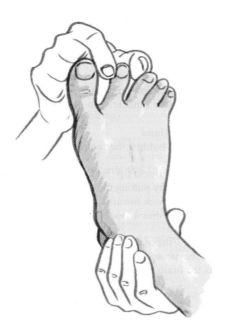

Tiny
As in caterpillar walk – a very small (almost imperceptible) forward caterpillar move.

Walking the Ridge
Achieved by caterpillar walk using a distinct downward pressure across the ridge of foot/hand where the toes/fingers join onto the foot/hand (eye/ear reflex). When toes are pushed away the ridge is visible. (Most pressure is on the lateral edge of the thumb).

Working Hand
The hand treating at any one time.

Zone Walking/Channel Clearing
To perform Zone Walking or Channel Clearing, caterpillar walk through the foot from heel to toe working from zone 1 to zone 5. Once the entire sole is treated then caterpillar down the dorsum, from toes to ankle.

Basic Finger/Thumb Technique/Caterpillar Walk

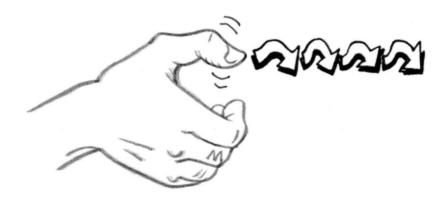

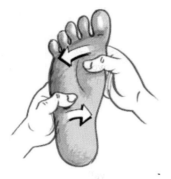

Criss-Cross Technique

Hook-In, Back Up Technique (Bee Sting Technique)

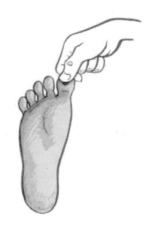

Pinch Push

45

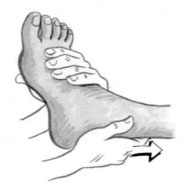

Slide Technique

Walking the Ridge

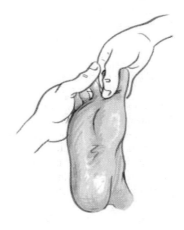

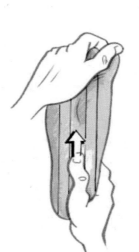

Zone Walking/Channel Clearing

46

ASPECTS OF TREATMENT

How Many Treatments:
This will vary according to a client's needs, reactions to treatment, feedback and overall benefit. In general, an experienced therapist would question the validity of the reflexology if no change has taken place after three treatments (however small those changes). The student would probably do six treatments to achieve a similar response.

Length of Each Session:
The treatment normally takes 45 minutes. In any event a one hour appointment should be made to allow for the comfort of the client, as reactions will vary from time to time and more relaxation strokes may have to be implemented. In order for the therapist to work within a commercially viable framework the client should be ready to leave within one hour of arrival, apart from the first session when one and a half hours would be more suitable in order to complete the consultation.

How Often to Treat:
Once a week is the general rule and it makes both practical and economic sense.

Adaptation of Treatment:
Treatments are given to meet the needs of the client. Whilst the average working time is 45 minutes, special needs such as age, condition, congestion, economic or physical circumstance and sensitivity levels may reduce the time or, with prior agreement with client and convenience of therapist, the time might actually be increased. A shorter, or lighter treatment would be more appropriate, for example, for a traumatised client prior/following major surgery, or for a client suffering from a bereavement.

Clients Treating Self, Between Treatments:
For those who are willing and able, then there is no reason why some reflex points cannot be demonstrated on the hand and guidance given in relation to pressure, frequency and number of times. Three to five reflexes seems to be enough to maintain interest. Emphasis should be placed on a client's own choice in this matter and it is not an absolute must to partake or continue.

Maintenance:
After the initial treatment return visits will vary according to the client's needs. Return visits will be variable: some weekly, monthly, bi-monthly, or even seasonal. The presenting condition and treatment review will play some part in the plan. The client must feel free to discontinue the treatment plan at any point and should not be pressurised into continuing or made to feel guilty for taking such a decision. The therapist must also feel free to discontinue treatment if he/she feels that to continue the treatment is not in the best interests of either the client or therapist.

Getting a Response:

Do not be discouraged if you do not get an excellent response straight away. A client very depleted of energy will usually take longer to respond than a more healthy fit person. Chronic conditions may take more treatments before a response of any significance is evident. All individuals are different and the response to treatment will be different. Some clients may become discouraged if there is not an immediate response, do not lose confidence. Concentrate on helping them to have a positive outlook. There is a lot going on under the surface. "Suddenly" things begin to change for what the client can accept as being for the better.

THE STRUCTURE OF THE FOOT

Feet act as effective shock absorbers. They are the foundation of the body and just like the foundations of any structure if these are faulty, serious defects can occur in any part of the structure. Foot disorders and inadequate foot wear that offers little support can result in spine, hip, knee and ankle problems. Tension on the spinal muscles can cause the cervical region (neck region) of the spine to tip forwards putting out the line of gravity (through the body). In turn this can lead to faulty posture. We are constantly using our backs getting up, sitting down, lifting, pulling and pushing and the force from this activity passes down the spine to the feet.

26 bones form the foot and ankle (one quarter of the bones in the human body).
33 joints hold the foot together and give flexibility.
Tendon The largest and strongest tendon is the Achilles which extends from the calf muscle to the heel.
Ligament The longest ligament is the Plantar Facia on the sole, stretching from the heel to the toes.
Nerve The main nerve to the foot is the posterior tibial, it passes down behind the inner ankle bone (medial malleolus). Each foot has thousands of nerve endings.
Blood Supply The main blood supply to the foot is the postior tibial artery, this runs behind the inner ankle along side the posterior tibial nerve.
Sweat Glands Each foot has about nine thousand sweat glands.
Forefoot This is composed of five toes called phalanges and their connecting long bones called metatarsals.
Phalanx Each toe has three small bones (phalanx), with the exception of the great toe (hallux) this has but two bones (phalanx).

Note
Within the tendon under the great toe are two small sesamoid bones hence sometimes we read that the foot has 28 bones.

Interphalangeal joints are formed between each of the toe bones.
Metatarsalphalangeal joints are formed where the toes and the metatarsals meet.
Midfoot This is formed by five irregular shaped bones namely –
1 cuboid, 3 cuneiform, 1 navicular and is connected to the forefoot and hindfoot by muscles and by the plantar facia.
Hindfoot This is formed by the calcaneus (heel bone) and the talus.
Ankle This is a complex mechanism. The true ankle joint is formed by the tibia (shin bone) coming together with the talus on the medial side forming the medial malleolous (ankle bone) and the fibula coming together with the talus on the lateral side to form the lateral malleolous (outside ankle bone). This joint is responsible for the up and down movement of the foot. The talus and calcaneus form a further joint which allows side to side movement of the foot.

BONES OF THE FOOT

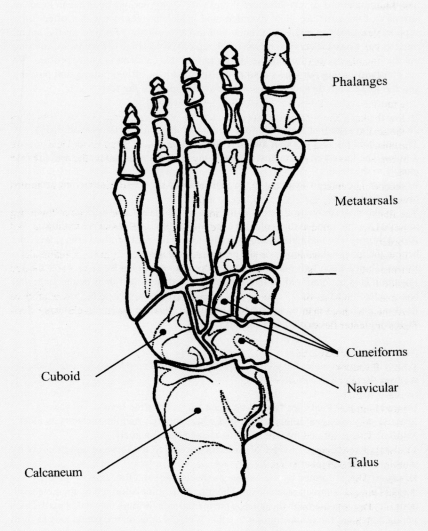

Phalanges

Metatarsals

Cuneiforms

Navicular

Cuboid

Talus

Calcaneum

MUSCLES OF THE FOOT

The Muscles -

> Help retain the arches
> Facilitate walking
> Enable the body to retain balance
> Give protective bulk to the foot

The muscles of the lower leg have an influence on the foot.

Below the knee all muscles are innervated by the tibial, or peroneal nerve (branches of the sciatic nerve).

The muscles of the leg produce downward movement at the ankle (flexion) and upward movement (extension or dorsiflexion) and they also help to maintain the arches of the foot.

A second movement below the ankle joint allows the sole of the foot to be turned inwards (inversion) and outwards (eversion).

The fibular (common peroneal) nerve winds around the neck of the fibula (lower leg bone) where it is superficial and liable to damage. This can sometimes result in foot disorders.

The stability and movement of the foot depends on muscles, ligaments and tendons. Extrinsic Muscles are so named because each muscle has an attachment that is located outside the foot.

The extrinsic muscles of the foot are multi- articular; they cross and therefore, produce movement at more than one articulation or joint. Each extrinsic muscle either dorsi flexes or planter flexes.

EXTRINSIC MUSCLES
Tibalis Posterior
Action- Plantar flexes, inverts foot
Nerve-   Tibial
Flexor Digitorum Longus
Action- Plantar flexes, inverts foot, flexes toes
Nerve-   Tibial
Flexor Hallucis Longus
Action- Plantar flexes, everts foot, flexes great toe
Nerve-   Tibial
Tibialis Anterior
Action- Dorsiflexes foot, inverts foot
Nerve-   Tibial
Extensor Digitorum Longus
Action- Dorsiflexes foot, everts foot, extends toes
Nerve-   Deep Peroneal

Extensor Hallucis Longus
Action- Dorsiflexes foot, everts foot, extends great toe
Nerve- Deep Peroneal
Peroneous Teritius
Action- Dorsiflexes foot, everts foot
Nerve- Deep Peroneal
Peroneus Longus
Action- Plantar Flexes foot, everts foot
Nerve- Superficial Peroneal
Peroneus Brevis
Action- Plantar flexes foot, everts foot
Nerve- Superficial Peroneal
Gastrocnemius
Action Plantar flexes foot, flexes leg
Nerve- Tibial
Soleus
Action- Planter flexes foot
Nerve- Tibial
Plantaris
Action- Plantar flexes foot
Nerve- Tibial

INTRINSIC MUSCLES
Extensor Digitorum Brevis (only dorsal muscle)
Action- Extends toes
Nerve- Deep Peroneal

PLANTAR MUSCLES
Abductor Hallicus   (first layer/superficial layer)
Action- Abducts great toe, flexes metatarsophalangeal joint
Nerve- Medial Plantar
Flexor Digitorum Brevis
Action- Flexes second through fifth toes
Nerve- Medial Plantar
Abductor Digiti minimi
Action- Abducts small toe, flexes small toe
Nerve- Lateral Plantar
Quadratus Plantae   (second layer)
Action- Flexes second through fifth toes
Nerve- Lateral Plantar
Lumbricals (4 small muscles)
Action- Extends second through fifth toes
Nerve- Medial and Lateral Plantar

Flexor Hallicus Brevis (third layer)
Action- Flexes great toe
Nerve- Medial Plantar
Adductor Hallicus Brevis
Action- Adducts great toe, flexes great toe
Nerve- Lateral Plantar
Flexor Digiti Minimi Brevis
Action- Flexes small toe
Nerve- Lateral Plantar
Dorsal Interosei
Action- Abducts toes, flexes proximal phlanges
Nerve- Lateral Plantar
Plantar Interosei
Action- Adducts third fourth and fifth toes and flexes proximal phlanges
Nerve- Lateral

THE ARCHES

The bones of the foot are so arranged as to produce three main arches:

The Medial Longitudinal Arch
This is the highest of the arches and is most visible on the inside of the foot. It is formed by:

6 bones – Talus, Calcaneus, Navicular, 3 Cuneiform bones, Metatarsals 1, 2, 3

Only the calcaneus (heel bone) and the distal end of the metatarsals should touch the ground.

The Lateral Longitudinal Arch
This is much less marked than the medial longitudinal arch and is composed of the:

Calcaneus
Cuboid
Metatarsals 4, 5

The Transverse Arch
This arch is formed by the:

Navicular
3 Cuneiform Bones
Cuboid
All 5 Metatarsals

The arches are not fixed and they flex as the weight of the body is transmitted to the ground. When the weight is removed they return to their original state.

The bones comprising the arches are held in position by ligaments and tendons. When these ligaments and tendons are weakened, the height of the medial longitudinal arch may decrease or 'fall' causing Flat Foot (*Pes Valgoplanus*).

ARCHES AND BONES OF THE FOOT

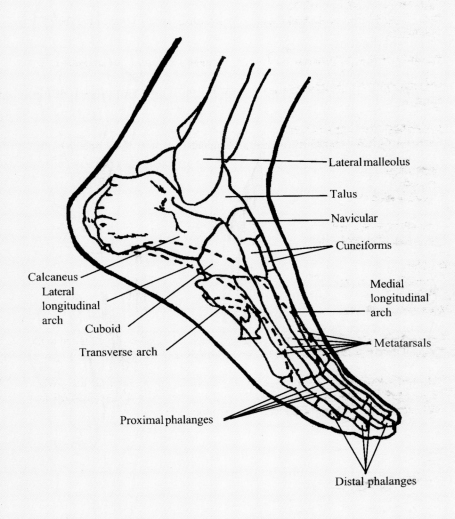

Lateral malleolus

Talus

Navicular

Cuneiforms

Medial longitudinal arch

Metatarsals

Calcaneus

Lateral longitudinal arch

Cuboid

Transverse arch

Proximal phalanges

Distal phalanges

WEIGHT BEARING

Weight bearing
bones of the foot

Outlined by triangle

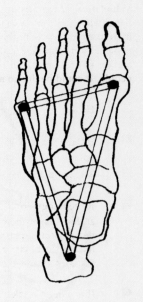

Cushioned weight
bearing area of the foot

Within outline

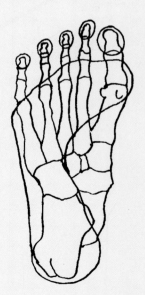

WHAT DO REACTIONS INDICATE?

What does sensitivity indicate?

Sensitivity indicates congestion/energy blockage, the more sensitive the area is, the more congested it is likely to be. Sensitivity and reactions will vary from person to person. I am sometimes asked, 'will all clients have sensitivity on most visits?' The answer is no, especially on the first or second visit, nothing much is felt by some people. It could be due to a number of factors, such as:

■ How a person perceives hurt/pain or sensitivity;

■ If there is a strong analgesic (pain killing) drug being taken;

■ The recipient may not be prepared to accept treatment at the moment;

■ Reflexology not being a cure all, may not be suitable for this particular person at this time in their life (a rare occurrence). However, in these cases, at least three or four treatments should be given before deciding on the suitability or likely effectiveness of Reflexology. Naturally client feed-back will also be a deciding factor in continuation or otherwise;

■ If a client has taken alcohol or recreational drugs (no matter how small the dose).

What are the Crystals (Gritty Bits)?

Uric acid and excess calcium are two of the waste products that build up in the body when the metabolism is not working according to plan. As a result of gravity, these deposits can be felt on the feet (usually near joints) like grains of sugar or sand. The little clumps can be broken down by the Reflexology technique. The broken down deposits are then carried by the blood and lymph flow to be eliminated by the body in the usual manner.

The Healing Reaction

As a result of the balancing effect of the treatment, symptoms may appear to worsen, but these are generally very short-lived before improving or disappearing. This means that the immune system is activated. The aftermath of these symptoms is to leave the client feeling good. Severe symptoms following a treatment can also lead to the client reconsidering further treatment. Reassurance, lighter pressure and perhaps a shorter treatment at the next visit should lessen the possibility of an acute reaction. Therapists should be mindful that such reactions may not be related to reflexology, but to other factors.

Note

Some therapists use the words 'healing crisis'. This suggests to me that the body has over-reacted to the treatment. Reasons are varied but may be due to client not having given sufficient information during consultation resulting in too much pressure or over treatment for that moment in time. Re-evaluation of the situation is necessary. The following treatment might be the Urgent Care Routine which would help the body to prepare for further treatment. (See Page 92)

WHAT IS ENERGY?
WHERE DOES IT COME FROM?

What Part Does It Have To Play In Reflexology?
Many cultures, including the Chinese believe the whole functioning of the body and mind depends on the normal flow of energy. Energy nourishes the organism, it is life's fuel. The energy central to holistic therapies usually referred to as *Chi, Ki* or *Prana* allows the body's integrated systems to achieve homeostasis. We can neither see nor feel energy in much the same way as we cannot see or feel radio waves or ultra violet. The energy in the body comes from the air we breathe and the food we eat. There is no doubt that when we eat nutritionally rich food we are also taking in strong energy. Strong energy also protects the body, acting as a defence system.

Western Approach
The language of Western medicine refers to this energy as having high resistance. When we are healthy and fit, if this energy (*chi* or *prana*) is weak, we in the West refer to it as lowered resistance/immunity, which can result in illness of body or mind. Whatever terminology we use, lowered energy, lowered immunity or lowered resistance, once illness has set in our inner resistance is of the greatest importance in restoring health. Interruptions in the flow of energy lead to an energy imbalance. This can cause disorders in parts of the body not apparently involved. Disorders and disease lead to further blocking of the energy flow. The body's immune system grows weak resulting in the possibility of multiple symptoms.

Reflexologists are aiming to strengthen and balance the energy flow by working with pressure on reflex points on the feet/hands. Many experienced reflexologists believe that reflex points are energy junctions on the zone pathway that respond to pressure.

Hippocrates found that a healing energy radiated from his hands when he was treating his patients. He wrote;

"It hath oft appeared, while I have been soothing a patient, as if there were some strange property in my hands to pull and draw away from the afflicted parts, aches and diverse impurities, by laying my hands upon the place and by extending fingers towards it".

Types of energy-related terms used in everyday language are:

Terminology	Meaning
Energy	The capacity to do work that is to put mass into motion.
Potential Energy	Inactive or stored energy, e.g. energy stored in a battery or a coiled spring.
Kinetic Energy	Energy of motion, e.g. any object in motion, a football, a molecule, a river.
Chemical Energy	The energy released or absorbed in the breaking apart or forming of chemicals, e.g. the building processes of the body, replacement of injured cells, construction of bone, or growth of hair and nails.
Food Energy	When foods are broken down the chemical energy given off is in a form that can be used for the building processes of the body.
Radiant Energy	Energy that travels in waves, e.g. heat and light. Others in everyday use are radio waves, microwaves (as in microwave ovens), infra-red waves (heat) ultra violet waves (can cause sunburn), x-rays and gamma rays (used in medical imaging).
Electric Energy	Results from the flow of electrons or other charged particles such as ions for example, impulses (action potential) in nerve and muscle cells.
Short Wave Length	Radiant waves of energy spaced close together
Long Wave Length	Radiant waves of energy spaced futher apart.

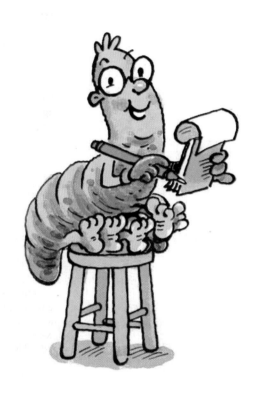

WHY REFLEXOLOGY?

■ Reflexology encourages a state of relaxation so that tension and the resultant toxicity held in the internal organs and in the muscle is released, thereby promoting healing.

■ Reflexology promotes homeostasis of all systems of the body through reduction of the effects of stress.

■ It has been estimated that seventy-five percent of disease is stress-related. As reflexology encourages relaxation this must be seen as a major benefit on the road to good health and maintenance.

■ The digestive system is encouraged to work to optimum efficiency. The passage of food and waste through the digestive tract is improved. Motility and tone of the smooth muscle of the stomach and intestine is increased. Hence through a more efficient digestive system energy is absorbed by the body. Every cell in the body benefits from the efficient distribution of nutrients initiated in the small intestine.

■ Reflexology encourages good circulation, hence the vessels of the heart receive optimum blood supply. Every cell in the body benefits from the efficient distribution of nourishment and waste elimination.

■ Through the thousands of nerve endings in the feet reflexology encourages and stimulates efficient flow of nerve impulses, i.e. nerve energy.

Note
Only second to the lips, is the tactile sensitivity of the feet and hands. These represent the greatest amount of tactile information (sensation) conveyed by the spinal nerves to the somatosensory area of the brain's cortex.

REFLEXOLOGY CAN...

- Reduce feelings of stress

- Calm and soothe

- Give the recipient a feeling of well-being

- Relax mind and body

- Encourage elimination

- Improve circulation

- Assist the body in maintaining a balanced state

CAUTIONS
AND
CONTRA INDICATIONS

CONDITION	CONTRA-INDICATION	CAUTION	RATIONALE
Acute, Undiagnosed Pain	X	X	It is recommended that a client should be referred to their GP for a medical diagnosis of their condition. If pain develops during treatment, emergency First Aid procedure applies.
AIDS/HIV and Hepatitis		X	Follow Standard Reflexology hygiene procedure. Light Pressure.
Aneurism - if known		X	Reflexology improves circulation
Arthritis with Inflammation or Pain.		X	Use a lighter pressure to accommodate client's needs.
Asthma		X	Should be familiar with standard first aid procedure.
Cancer - including Blood and Bone Cancer		X	Understand the medical treatment and the likely reactions of treatment in relation to pressure. Awareness of low platelet count and potential bruising is important. It is recommended that practitioners undertake further training prior to treating in this sector.

CONDITION	CONTRA-INDICATION	CAUTION	RATIONALE
Cellulitis	**X** Severe Cases	**X**	Use light pressure; direct pressure on affected area is likely to be painful and therefore not appropriate. In severe cases, do not treat the affected area. Treat hands to avoid contra-indication.
Contagious or Notifiable Disease	**X**		Risk of infection and cross-infection makes this a contra-indication.
Diabetes		**X**	Light pressure should be used as client's healing potential may be impaired. They may have lessened sensitivity, peripheral neuropathy, finer skin, bruise easily or be prone to ulceration on legs and feet. A treatment using appropriate pressure will be of benefit. (In severe cases diabetes may result in Gangrene this is contra-indicated - obtain immediate medical attention).

66

CONDITION	CONTRA-INDICATION	CAUTION	RATIONALE
Drugs or Alcohol Abuse - patient out of control or mental state appears unstable	**X** If lacking the skills/facilities to cope		If a client presents for treatment under the influence, there may be a safety risk to the practitioner. If a client who is dependant on alcohol or other substance presents for treatment and is *not* under the influence, then the practitioner should be able to proceed with caution. Proceed in a similar way if the client is in recovery. There may be risk of severe reaction/healing response. Alcoholic seizure may occur. Practitioners should undertake appropriate training.
Epilepsy		**X**	Have an understanding of the condition, how to prevent injury in the event of a seizure and how to administer First Aid.
Imminent Medical Tests or Procedures	**X** Depends on the test	**X**	The results *might* not be representative and overview may be distorted by the improvements resulting from reflexology treatment.

CONDITION	CONTRA-INDICATION	CAUTION	RATIONALE
Injury to the Feet		X	Practitioners should be able to treat in order to accommodate the client's needs. Use hand reflexology, etc. or avoid affected area.
Heart Condition, Unstabilised	X Depends on Condition/Inst-ability	X	If a client is unstable then they are probably under the care of the hospital. Treatment during this time would only be possible with consent, adequate supervision and the emergency facilities to hand.
Medication		X	When, for a serious condition, the benefits resulting from reflexology might alter the amount of medication required, treatment should be carried out with the cooperation of the prescribing doctor. Be aware of side effects of drugs, e.g. steroids, bruising etc.
Menstruation		X	Probably best to avoid giving a treatment during a heavy flow. If treating however, use a lighter pressure at this time. Reflexology can help such a client.

CONDITION	CONTRA-INDICATION	CAUTION	RATIONALE
Osteoporosis		X	Be aware of the fragility of a client's bones and that a lighter pressure is more appropriate.
Phlebitis		X	Use a lighter pressure and no direct pressure on affected area as it is likely to be painful. In severe cases it may be impossible to work the affected area, though unlikely on the feet. Use hand reflexology.
Surgery		X	*Before surgery*: Practitioner could inform client that treatment may provoke a healing response - especially with first treatment or with patients who are very sick. Treatment can help to prepare for surgery. *After surgery*: Treatment can be very helpful post-operatively once client is signed off or with permission from the surgeon.

CONDITION	CONTRA-INDICATION	CAUTION	RATIONALE
Pregnancy		**X**	Practitioners should remember two lives are involved! Some practitioners may choose to avoid giving treatment for fear of litigation. Some clients claim reflexology has helped during their entire pregnancy. Working with clients who are pregnant: It is strongly recommended that practitioners undertake further training to optimise support for the client. Be aware of danger signs.
Thrombosis/DVT - If known * (*Frequently clients do not know they have a DVT)	**X**	**X**	When the client has a DVT diagnosis, treatment is contra-indicated until stabilised and then the therapist must proceed with caution. *After flying*: Check for signs of thrombosis, in some cases both therapist and client may prefer to defer treatment for at least 72 hours.

CONDITION	CONTRA-INDICATION	CAUTION	RATIONALE
Thyroidism, Hyper and Hypo		X	Client's medication may need to be adjusted in cooperation with their GP.
Varicose Veins, Severe		X	Direct pressure on affected area should be avoided.
Verrucae		X	Area should be covered or avoided and client referred for treatment. Treat corresponding reflex on hand.
Vaccination		X	May bring about a severe healing response. Wait at least 72 hours.

These contra indications are written with the qualified therapist in mind. Students should be guided by their tutor during their initial training. Some listings under caution will be classified as contra indications until competency is established.

For the student initial practise should be on healthy individuals. Those conditions listed under cautions should only be attempted when pressure, rhythm and holds are perfected and the condition fully understood.

REACTIONS TO REFLEXOLOGY TREATMENT

It is impossible to predict how any person's body will react or respond to a reflexology treatment. The following paragraphs outline the more general type of reactions that might occur. Most of these reactions relate in some way to the release of toxins into the system and how the body copes with them.

A high percentage of clients have no adverse reaction, just a steady improvement of the symptoms, leading to a measurable relief. Some have total cessation of symptoms, with the acute condition tending to respond more quickly than the chronic condition.

Cramp, crawling, electric shock, feeling warm, feeling cold on corresponding side or opposite side: all these reactions are normal and in response to nerve stimulation.

Long Term Illnesses
Serious and long term illness can be very debilitating to the body and result in poor elimination and detoxification by the dedicated organs, such as the liver and the kidneys.

Medication
Drugs may accumulate in the body because the liver cannot process and break down these substances efficiently.

Elimination
If the kidneys are not working to optimum efficiency they in turn cannot eliminate the toxins quickly enough and they may re-enter the blood stream. These clients may have a strong healing reaction.

Clients who are Unwell
Always approach the unwell client and those on long term medication with a lighter pressure and consider a straight forward treatment of all reflexes without supporting additional treatment of reflexes until you can assess outcomes.

Urgent Care Routine
The therapist may consider that the *'Renée Tanner Urgent Care Routine'* might be the most suitable option for the introduction to reflexology for some clients, e.g. those who are frail through illness or the very young, who may not be able to deal with a strong reaction to treatment. However there are others who benefit from this 'urgent care' treatment but are unable to tolerate a full treatment due, for example, to incapacitation or strong medication. They could gain more therapeutic value from the session by the addition of treatment to the reflexes related to a specific condition.

The *'Urgent Care Routine'* is described in full on page 92.

Listings for specific conditions can be found on page 83.

Some of the reactions that might happen during treatment:

■ **A feeling of being very cold.**
Use a lighter than normal pressure. Cover client with a light blanket.
Lowered blood pressure – letting go of deep emotions.

■ **Changes in expression.**
Discuss* – happy, sad, pain.

■ **Crying, groaning, laughing, sighing or singing.**
Discuss* – a sign of emotional release

■ **Gestures of pain.**
Discuss* – sensitive reflex, cramp, discomfort, not related to the therapy.

■ **Profuse sweating on the palms of the hands.**
Discuss* – usually a sign of release, possibly emotional.

■ **Visible contraction of the muscles.**
Discuss* – pain, discomfort, mental imagery.

To calm and relax a stressed client
Speak in a calm voice while gently effleuraging the whole foot. The effleurage can be alternated with a diaphragm and solar plexus treatment and/or stroking or just stop and hold. Alternatively the therapist should also be aware that reactions unrelated to Reflexology could well occur in the clinic; for example, a heart attack or asthmatic attack. It is for this reason it is generally accepted that all practising therapists should hold a valid Certificate in First Aid.

Note
Client's blood pressure usually drops a little during treatment not only due to the beneficial effect of the treatment but also to the quiet, relaxed treatment atmosphere which helps to reduce stress.

* Discuss is used in this context as 'an exchange of information'.

Reactions that may occur between treatment visits

These can sometimes involve temporary discomfort or pain:

Elimination:

- Increase in urination.

- Increase in bulk, volume and frequency of the stool.

- Increase in nasal secretions.

- Increase of, or the appearance of vaginal discharge.

Generally:

- Toothache, usually due to tooth decay or gum infections.

- Feeling very tired. The body is working overtime to bring about healing and elimination.

- Feeling very sleepy. Relaxation, letting go.

- Feeling wonderful. Restored energy.

Clients may explain how, for example, they caught a cold last week after they had received a treatment. They will sometimes go on to express their fears of getting a cold, etc, if they have more treatments. It is worthwhile taking the time to explain to the client that all illness is preceded by an incubation period which may last for days, or much longer, before the illness becomes apparent. Reflexology will not cause a cold. All reactions such as those described are due to the body's own healing and elimination processes.

All clients who react in an unusual way, or give the therapist grounds to suspect a serious illness must be referred to their own doctor. The therapist can always contact the client's doctor by letter explaining his/her fears (the client's written consent is required). Where a client is under medical investigation, is receiving specialised treatment, or is pregnant they should be advised to notify their medical team that they are receiving reflexology.

JOINT LOOSENING EXERCISES TO PRACTISE BEFORE YOU START

1) Stand with outstretched arms in front. Open and close hands ten times.

2) Stand still, holding arms outstretched as in the previous movement. Bend hand up and down from wrist ten times slowly, ten times fast.

3) Extend the arms to the side. Rotate wrist rapidly in a clockwise direction ten times. Repeat the movement in an anti-clockwise direction ten times.

4) Remain standing. Extend arms out to the side and push backwards twice. Bring arms to the front. Stretch out and push forward twice. Repeat complete movement ten times.

5) Stretch arms out in front, fingers pointing straight ahead, little finger side of hand towards the floor, thumb towards the ceiling. Hold fingers slightly apart. Now move hand from wrist up and down slowly at first, gradually getting faster.

6) Stretch arms out in front. Close hand into fist, thumb on outside of fist. Now throw your hands open. Repeat ten times.

7) Sit down and relax for a few minutes then bring your hands across in front of you. Close fingers into palm, but leave thumb free. Try to make your thumbs bow to each other by bending the first joint (joint nearest nail). Repeat ten times.

8) Remain seated and this time try the movement by using your index finger (finger next to thumb) and remember to repeat ten times.

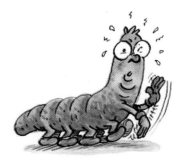

75

MASSAGE/RELAXATION TECHNIQUES

In the interest of clarity of description and to avoid any confusion about reflexology there are some therapists that will differentiate between massage and relaxation techniques. In reality this is related to the language used, rather than the description of the movement. Massage techniques are used to bring about relaxation, hence the phrase 'relaxation techniques'.

The movements are employed prior to and on completion of the reflexology sequence and some movements can be interspersed with the reflexology treatment, especially when there is a high degree of sensitivity or stress. There are approximately three thousand movements for the massage therapist to draw on for this purpose, however here I will suggest a selection that would be appropriate for relaxation. When you are familiar with and have perfected the techniques described here then if needs be you can expand your skills in the future by practicing the selection on page 131. In my opinion it is best to keep to about six movements in any one treatment and repeat a couple where necessary.

Movement 1
Place both hands side by side, on the top of the foot. Slide down the foot to the ankle. Part your hands so one is on the inner ankle and the other on the outer ankle, then massage around each ankle using two middle fingers. Do the movement 4 times.

Movement 2
Cup the heel in one hand and wrap the other hand around the foot with the thumb on the sole and fingers on the dorsum (top). Slowly rotate the foot, firstly in a clockwise movement, then in an anticlockwise movement. Do the movement 3 times in each direction.

Movement 1

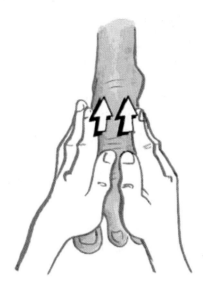

Movement 2

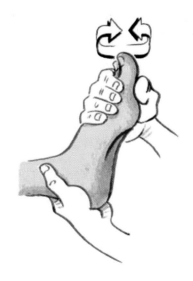

Movement 3

Put pad of hands (part below fingers = pad) one on either side of the edge of the foot, just below the big toe (distal) with your fingers pointing up in the air. Push the medial aspect (big toe side) away from you while gently pulling the lateral aspect (little toe side) towards you, then repeat the movement in the opposite direction. Do the movement 3 times in each direction.

Movement 4

Wrap the fingers of both hands around the dorsum (top) of the foot, one hand higher up the foot than the other. Put your thumbs resting in a similar position on the sole. Now use your thumbs to stroke in and out across the sole. Cover the whole sole in this manner, working down firstly from below the toes to the heel then back up again. Do the movement twice in each direction.

Movement 3

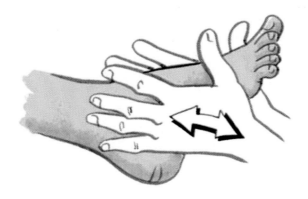

Movement 4

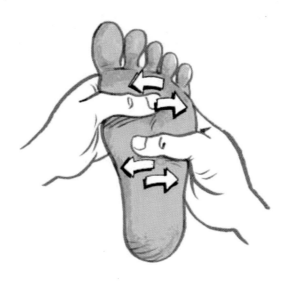

79

Movement 5

Support the foot by resting the outer edge on one hand. Use the heel (thenar eminence) of the working hand to stroke down the inside of the foot, from big toe to heel. Then work in the opposite direction. **Note**: follow the curves of the *bone*, do not work on the sole. Do the movement 3 times in each direction.

Movement 6

Wrap the fingers of both hands around the dorsum (top) of the foot, one hand higher up the foot than the other. Put your thumbs resting in a similar position on the sole, pull up all the way to the base of the toes. At the toes turn your thumbs upwards and spread the toes gently apart by sliding your fingers along the backs.

Movement 7 and Movement 8 (Repeats)

For number 7, repeat movement number 2, rotating the foot. For movement number 8, repeat movement number 1, sliding down the foot and around the ankles.

Movement 5

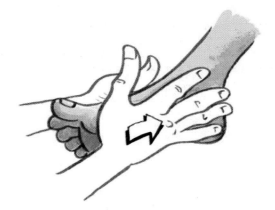

Movement 6

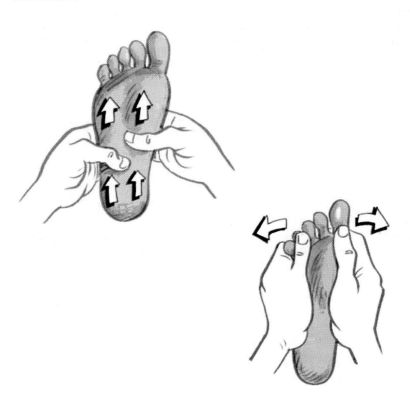

SELF HELP TREATMENT/ GUIDELINES FOR THE PROFESSIONAL THERAPIST

The following list will be helpful for those who wish to give a self help treatment. The overall results will be more successful when coupled with a zone walk/channel clearing sequence, prior to and on completion of treating the specific reflex.

While a self treatment will help to alleviate symptoms it is not a substitute for treatment from a professional therapist who will treat all reflexes in accordance with a client's needs. The professional is also trained to recognise reflex reaction and to consider whether more or less treatment would be appropriate. The therapist will also refer the client to a medical practitioner or therapist with the appropriate skills.

As previously stated, self treatment while being helpful will never be as beneficial as a treatment given by another, as it is impossible to achieve the same degree of relaxation and equally as difficult to perceive one's own bodily reactions. Self help treatment is more usually performed on the hands due to ease of access.

LIST OF DISORDERS

The professional therapist can use the following list in support of a full treatment.

There are a number of areas that, when focussed on during a treatment routine will help bring about a good response in those clients presenting either with symptoms or with a diagnosis of a particular disorder or disease.

The following list is not inclusive of all conditions that could be treated with reflexology (that is a book in itself) neither is it intended to show all reflex points relevant to each condition as symptoms/conditions may have a number of causes. What is listed here is the reflexes most likely to be beneficial to the relevant condition. To be inclusive of all reflexes that would be appropriate to treat for the relevant condition would in effect be suggesting a full treatment routine.

ACNE
Pituitary
Lymphatics Head/Neck/Thoracic
Liver
Kidney
Adrenal
Ovary (female) Testes and Prostate (male)

ALLERGIES
Eyes (if problem)
Lymphatics Head/Neck/Thoracic
Liver
Spleen
Adrenal
Small Intestine
Colon

ANEMIA
Liver
Spleen
Spine
Lungs
Sternum

ANKLES

Heart
Kidney
Adrenal
Sciatic
Inguinal lymphatics and spleen

ARM PITS (AXILLARY)

Advise the client to have any abnormalities in this area checked by a medical practitioner (GP)
Shoulder
Spine
Lymphatics Head/Neck/Thoracic

ARTHRITIS

Head/Neck
Shoulder/Arm/Knee/Hip
Thyroid
Parathyroid
Spine
Kidney
Adrenals
Lymphatics (all) including spleen

ASTHMA

Head/Brain/Face
Pituitary
Thyroid
Lymphatics including the spleen
Lungs
Adrenals

BACKACHE

Thyroid
Parathyroid
Spine
Shoulder/Arm/Knee/Hip
Kidney
Lymphatics (all)

BLADDER DISORDERS

Pituitary
Parathyroid
Liver
Spleen
Kidney/Ureter Tubes/Bladder
Adrenals

BLOOD PRESSURE

Pituitary
Thyroid
Parathyroid
Heart
Kidney
Adrenal

BREAST PROBLEMS PRIOR TO MENSTRUATION

Pituitary
Breast
Kidney
Adrenal
Ovary
Lymphatics Head/Neck/Thoracic

BRONCHITIS

Face
Neck
Lung
Adrenal
Lymphatics Head/Neck/Thoracic

BURSITIS

Parathyroid
Shoulder/Arm/Knee/Leg/Hip
Kidney/Ureters/Bladder
Adrenal
Lymphatics (all)

CHOLESTROL

Thyroid
Liver/Gall Bladder
Stomach
Pancreas
Heart -treat within professional full treatment routine, not within this section

COLD

It would be advisable for the therapist to wear a mask when treating this client. The urgent care routine supported with treatment of the lymphatics and adrenals would be sufficient during a cold

CONSTIPATION

Liver/Gall Bladder
Stomach
Small Intestine
Spine
Adrenal
Colon
Lymphatics (all)

CRAMP LEG

Thyroid
Parathyroid
Knee/Leg/Hip
Spine
Sciatic nerve

DIGESTIVE PROBLEMS

Head
Oesophagus
Stomach/Pancreas/Duodenum
Liver
Small Intestine
Lymphatics (all)
Colon

EAR DISORDERS

Mastoid Process
Face/ Front of Neck
Sinuses/Cranial Nerves
Ear
Eustachian Tube
Shoulder
Adrenal

EYE DISORDERS

Head/Brain/Face
Cranial Nerves
Eye
Kidney
Adrenal
Cervical Spine

FEMALE and MALE DISORDERS (related to reproductive system)

Hypothalamus/Pituitary
Thyroid
Liver
Kidney
Adrenal
Uterus/Prostate
Ovary/Testicle
Fallopian Tube/Vas Deferens

FLATULANCE (wind)

Stomach/Duodenum/Pancreas
Liver
Small Intestine
Colon/Ileocaecal Valve
Lymphatica (all)

FORGETFULNESS (stress related)

Head/Brain
Hypothalamus/Pituitary
Thyroid
Parathyroid
Spine
Shoulder
Adrenal

GALL BLADDER DISORDERS

Parathyroid
Gall Bladder
Liver
Kidney
Small Intestine
Colon

GOUT

Pituitary
Thyroid
Parathyroid
Kidney
Adrenal
Small Intestine
Lymphatics (all)
Colon

HAY FEVER

Pituitary
Face
Eyes
Lungs
Adrenal
Lymphatics Head/Neck

HEADACHE

Head/Brain/Pituitary
Cranial Nerves/Sinuses
Eyes/Ears
Stomach/Pancreas
Liver/Gall Bladder
Kidney
Shoulder
Spine
Adrenal
Lymphatics Head/Neck

HEART

All heart conditions should be checked by a medical practitioner (GP)
Urgent Care routine is most suitable (See page 188)
Professional therapists treat within routine if medically suitable

INSOMNIA

Head/Brain
Spine
Shoulder
Kidneys
Adrenal

KIDNEY DISORDERS

Kidney disorders need to be investigated by a medical practitioner (GP)
Pituitary
Thyroid
Kidney/Ureter/Bladder
Adrenal
Spine

LIVER DISORDERS

Liver disorders need to be investigated by a medical practitioner (GP)
Thyroid
Parathyroid
Liver
Gall Bladder
Spleen
Kidneys
Small Intestine
Colon
Lymphatics

LUNG DISORDER

Neck
Trachea
Lungs
Spleen
Liver
Adrenal
Spine

NAUSEA

Head/Brain
Cranial Nerves
Ear/ Balance
Stomach
Liver
Kidney
Small Intestine
Colon

SCIATICA

Adrenal
Sciatic Nerve
Spine
Hip
Colon

SINUSITIS

Pituitary
Head/Brain/Face
Cranial Nerves/Sinuses
Teeth/Gums
Eyes
Small Intestine
Kidney
Lymphatics Head/Neck
Colon

SKIN DISORDERS

Pituitary
Thyroid
Parathyroid
Adrenal
Ovary Female /Testes Male
Liver
Kidney
Small Intestuine
Lymphatics (all)
Colon

STRESS

Head/Brain
Cranial Nerves
Front/Back Neck
Thyroid/Parathyroid
Lungs
Stomach
Spine
Shoulder
Adrenals

VARICOSE VEINS

Lungs
Heart
Knee/Leg/Hip
Kidney
Adrenals
Small Intestine
Large Intestine
Lymphatics (all)

URGENT CARE ROUTINE SELF-HELP TREATMENT AND PROFESSIONAL GUIDE

The following reflexology routine is simple to perform and offers a general boost in helping to bring the body back to a state of homeostasis. This routine is known as the *'Renee Tanner Urgent Care Routine'*. It can be performed on its own or with the addition of treatment to the reflexes that are known to be out of order. The treatment sequence is also used by professional therapists in situations when and where, in the judgement of the professional a full treatment would not be appropriate.

The first thing to do would be to practice and perfect some relaxing massage movements and to use these before and after the reflexology routine. You could choose from those on page 131.

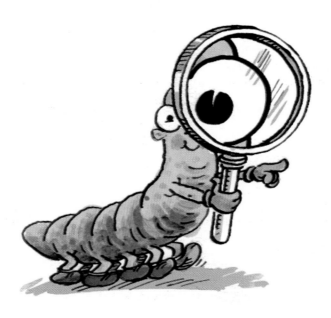

URGENT CARE REFLEXOLOGY

1. *Diaphragm line caterpillar walk, Solar Plexus pressure:*
   To encourage relaxed breathing, elimination of carbon dioxide and the uptake of oxygen.

   (See page 144)

2. *Zone Walk/Zone Clearing:*
   This treatment will cover all reflexes in a gentle way, encouraging the energy to flow freely all around the body. Make sure you cover the entire foot (remember between toes). This may take more than five walks depending on the size of the foot. Treat the hand in a similar way. The zone walk can be done between one and three times depending on client tolerance.

3. *Head, Brain and Face caterpillar walk:*
   To awaken senses and prepare for reception and delivery of messages.

   (See page 148)

4. *Spine caterpillar walk:*
   To clear nerve pathways to all areas of the body. Due to the huge nerve pathways treatment of this reflex will indirectly give a general body treatment.

   (See page 207)

   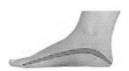

5.   *Kidney*

Three gentle presses to aid filtration and improve elimination.

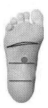

6.   *Colon*

To encourage elimination. Can be treated between 1-5 times depending on tolerance level of client. (See page 216)

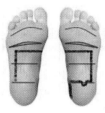

For the more adventurous self help therapist, with time, mobility and agility the reflexes listed on page 234 and relative to a specific disorder could be incorporated and treated as appropriate. However for both the professional and self help therapist it might be good practice not to add any further reflex treatment until the outcomes of the first treatment can be assessed and evaluated.

PROFESSIONALISM

This outlines what should be considered as the general behaviour of the therapist:

- Always wear a clean and appropriate uniform. Dresses/skirts should be below the knee.

- Wear the badge of a professional organisation.

- Talk to the client. Do not gossip or ask irrelevant, intrusive or personal questions.

- Give each client your undivided attention.

- Do not discuss one client with another.

- Do not talk about your own personal problems or life style that is not what the client is paying for.

- Always have client consideration, never dictate to the client.

ETHICS

This outlines what could be considered as the general principles of the therapist:

- All professional therapists incur an obligation to uphold the dignity of the profession and they shall at all times act honourably towards their clients and fellow practitioners.

- Professional therapists shall at all times honour the code of confidentiality in relation to their clients.

- Professional therapists will refrain from criticising the work of other professional practitioners, both medical and complementary.

- Professional practitioners should at all times (on duty and in social life) behave in a manner becoming to their profession and not behave in a way likely to bring embarrassment upon themselves or their profession.

- Professional practitioners undertake to confine treatments to within their skills and capabilities.

- Professional practitioners undertake not to offer cures for specific conditions.

- No therapist who is not a registered medical practitioner shall accept clients for medical diagnosis or treatment.

- Professional therapists undertake not to poach the clients of his or her employer.

PERSONAL HYGIENE

- Take a daily bath or shower.

- Prevent body odour by using a deodorant.

- Use a mouthwash to prevent bad breath.

- Clean teeth twice daily. Have regular dental checks.

- Have a clean handkerchief in case of the necessity to cough or sneeze and use it when necessary. Do not sneeze or cough over others.

- Wear clean clothes and underwear daily.

- Don't forget the socks, stockings or tights. They need changing at least once a day.

- Keep hair clean and tidy. Make sure it does not fall onto your face when your head is bent, as this can obscure the client's view. Most people would prefer to see our faces when talking to us.

- Keep nails short and, like the whole hand, impeccably clean.

- Wash hands before and after each treatment.

- Wash hands after using the toilet.

- Wear a clean uniform or coat. It looks professional.

- Wear clean shoes.

- You must be able to take care of yourself, before you attempt to take care of others.

You are offering a personal service where you are in very close proximity to others and your odour can be offensive to them. So if you smoke, drink alcohol, coffee or tea, or enjoy spicy food, remember the smell can linger, not just on your breath but some of these may be smelled on your clothes as well.

It is also worth bearing in mind that perfumes and aftershaves need to be used sparingly. The client might not share your love for a particular make or brand.

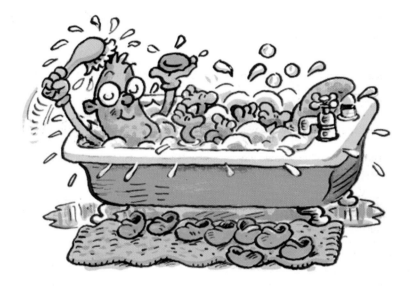

HYGIENE AT WORK

Hygiene is of the utmost importance in any treatment. When dealing with feet it is worth bearing in mind that the possibility of infection and contagion is always present. Conditions such as Athlete's Foot (*Tinea Pedis*), fungal infections of the nail and Verruca (a flat wart) are but a few examples of contagious conditions.

1. The therapist's hands must be washed before and after each treatment.

2. A paper towel should be used to dry the feet if they have been washed.

3. Rest client's feet on a paper towel during treatment.

4. Cover knee and foot rest with tissue. If tissue is not used then the covers must be changed after each client and washed before any further use.

5. Application of all solutions to the feet should be with cotton wool, tissue or antiseptic wipe. Clean cotton wool, tissue or wipe to be used for each foot.

6. Sterilise wash bowl with liquid disinfectant after each use.

7. All disposable material should be placed in a pedal bin immediately after use.

8. Have a pair of disposable gloves nearby for emergencies (e.g. athlete's foot requiring a closer examination).

9. The clinic should have a pedal bin. At the end of the day waste should be placed in a plastic bag and sealed ready for refuse collection. Waste stored outside should be placed in a bin with a lid on. This prevents the plastic bag from being destroyed by animals, leaving waste and litter on the ground.

10. Make sure working area is clean and surroundings pleasant. Daily floor and surface washing is essential as is disinfecting of couch, stool, clients' chairs and coat hooks, etc.

11. Do not smoke or allow client/patient to smoke during treatment or in the treatment area.

12. Check toilet and wash room following each client, ensure floor, sink and toilet is clean and that there is sufficient soap, toilet tissue and hand wipes. If electrical hand dryer is used, check regularly that it is working properly.

13. Blood spills should be wiped up immediately (**wear disposable gloves**). Pour bleach or similar recommended liquid on to the area. Leave for 5 minutes then wash the area with warm soapy water.

14. Blood soiled tissue should be placed in a yellow bag (or colour as sanctioned by the health authority/environmental authority of your country of residence). Collection and disposal of this bag must be agreed via local environmental health department or specialised agency.

THE 7 'C's OF TREATMENT

Caution
When a treatment can be given exercising caution and/or adaptation.

Communication Skills
The transmitting and receiving of information. Active listening is non-verbal communication, it is also, when we are silent. Non-verbal skills are methods of communication through our actions, be aware of proximity (personal space), orientation, posture, gestures, facial expressions, eye contact, touch and privacy. Active verbal communication means that the therapist may use questioning techniques. Be aware of certain types of questions: open, leading and probing; and of types of responses. For example therapists might use reflective, re-stating, clarifying and summarising responses.

Confidentiality
An agreement not to repeat what has been heard, said or written outside the client – practitioner situation ('outside these four walls'). Some clinics have a policy of sharing information regarding clients. Permission should be sought from the client and a signature obtained beforehand. Some clinics have a policy of storing information where the reception is located and where other staff may possibly have access to client information. Again the client's written consent must be obtained beforehand. In neither of the above two situations is confidentiality being maintained by the therapist though there may be a clinic policy in place with regard to confidentiality. In all cases in the UK the policy must meet with the data protection regulations.

Consent
Agreement between two or more people to an action taking place or the recognition of a verbal or written communiqué as being accurate. In reflexology this is generally a signature of the client agreeing to the accuracy of the information given, in relation to health, and the therapist's signature in agreement to confidentiality.

Consultation
A means through verbal communication, visual observation and listening skills to assess the client's needs, wants and expectations. To give verbal feedback, for example to explain therapy limitations and procedures.

Contra-Indications
Situations that arise in health or otherwise that suggest treatment is not suitable at this time and therefore should not take place.

Counselling Skills

A process whereby a person, in an understanding atmosphere, enables another, by purposeful conversation, to explore and make his own decisions given the choices available to him. Reflexologists have a basic training in listening skills and as such are not generally classified as counsellors unless they have undertaken a separate training of a minimum of two years in this specific subject.

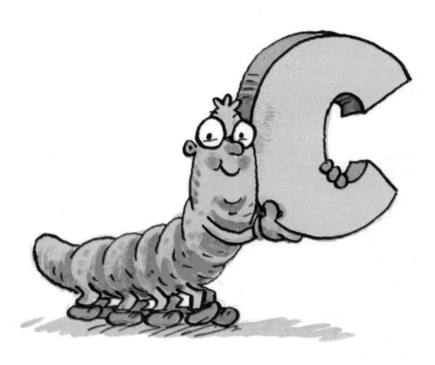

PROFESSIONAL ASSESSMENT PRIOR TO TREATMENT

Your senses and observations should come into play in order to access the client's needs prior to treatment. This assessment does not begin with the initial writing of the consultation but rather when you first hear the voice on the telephone and also when your client first comes into your view. Use your senses. You are in possession of a very powerful tool. Do note that not all that is spoken will tell you all that is really being said.

When the client arrives:

LOOK at body language, demeanour, self care (grooming), facial expression, skin colour and eyes ('the windows of the soul') and what they are telling you.

LISTEN to voice, tone, pitch, pace, power; both when on the telephone and when face to face.

SMELL natural body odour, poor hygiene, breath – cigarette smoke, alcohol.

SHOES – make an observation of the shoes that are worn, as some foot and leg complaints may be directly related. High heels put pressure on the toes and restrict flexibility.

Shoes that are not a snug fit may cause the foot to slip forward, damaging the toes and toe nails. This complaint is not uncommon in runners and those involved in playing racket sports. Ill fitting shoes may cause overstrain on the mechanics of the foot resulting in problems of the ankle joint, Achilles tendon and calf muscle (*gastrocnemius*).

Shoes with worn down heels, especially to one side, may indicate a possible hip/knee problem on that side.

Changing the heel shape and/or height may result in headaches due to the change in posture alignment which may cause pressure on the nerves at the back of the neck (in the cervical area).

CLIENTS WITH SPECIAL NEEDS AND CONSIDERATIONS

Age	Digit	Pressure	Treatment	Stroke
Neonate	index, middle or little finger	very light	zone walk once	i) diaphragm and solar plexus ii) head/brain (big toe) iii) spine iv) area of problem
Infant	index, middle finger or thumb	light	zone walk once or twice, depending on size and state of health. Once if ill. Progress to full treatment as time & child's tolerance allows.	i) diaphragm and solar plexus ii) head/brain iii) spine iv) area of problem
Child under 16 years	Either finger or thumb, depending on age	Adjust according to size/stature & feedback from child	Will depend on reason for visit & child's assessed tolerance level. Aim for a full treatment, if in doubt treat initially as for an infant, progressing to full treatment on a future visit, once time is given to investigate concerns.	Explain what you are doing to both parent and child, self help should be explained to child and confirmed with parent/ guardian.

Teenagers

Boys: Be aware of possible concerns: weight, skin disorders, e.g. acne, eczema, foot fungus, self-consciousness, shyness, vulnerability. Professionalism must be uppermost in the mind.

Girls: Be aware of the possible concerns above plus additional issues: eating disorders, menstrual disorders and pregnancy. Professionalism must be uppermost in the mind and a consciousness of the client gender and vulnerability of age.

Cancer

Reflexology is considered an ideal treatment to support patients. Treating cancer patients requires a firm foundation to work confidently in this specialised area. The therapist needs the knowledge and skill to deliver appropriate treatment and to effectively address patient and family queries and concerns. The cancer centre/team should be aware the patient is receiving reflexology. C.P.D (continuing professional development) is strongly recommended.

Diabetes

Clients with diabetes should be treated with a lighter pressure than might be considered appropriate for the size of the foot. Some diabetics may have lessened sensitivity to touch, skin is fine, they bruise easily and have a slow healing rate. Thoroughly check their feet for cuts and grazes at each session. Shoes, socks, stockings and tights should be seam free (see note on Drugs/Medication).

Clients with Disabilities

There may be a need to adapt working area, pressure and technique. Treat hands instead of feet or one of each. Be aware of possible limitations of movement that may have less obvious signs, e.g. an immovable knee joint that requires the leg to be kept straight all the time. Back problems that reduce the ability to get onto a treatment couch. Sciatic or hip disorders that reduce comfortable sitting time to a maximum of 15/20 minutes. If a client is confined to bed, adaptation of the client's position may be necessary. Nerve damage may mean a lessening of sensitivity. Be aware of pressure and the possibility of skin or vascular damage. If the client cannot weight bear, do not lift unless you are qualified to do so.

Drugs/Medication

Recreational and medicinal self-prescribed or medically prescribed drugs can reduce sensitivity to your touch, as can alcohol and nicotine. Those clients on sedatives or psychotrophic drugs may have a slower response to both touch and verbal communication. However as reflexology begins to take effect, balancing the body, it may be possible with the support and supervision of the client's medical doctor to reduce the medication. Similarly diabetic clients may be able to reduce medication, but again only under strict medical supervision. Diabetic clients should be advised to monitor their blood sugar levels very carefully. The therapist should use lighter pressure.

Elderly Clients
Listen carefully to needs and be aware that the client might have hearing, sight, speech, or mobility impairment. Take extra time to explain the treatment and ensure the client understands. Use less pressure and possibly shorten the duration of the treatment. Make sure the client is physically well supported with cushions and be aware of brittle bones, crepey skin, vascular disturbance, nerve damage and reduced adipose tissue. Give assistance with coat, shoes, etc.

Epilepsy
A client with Epilepsy will benefit from a full treatment. Pressure should be more gentle on the reflexes of the head, neck and cervical spine. The liver reflex could have extra treatment (see notes on reactive liver reflex in full routine). Be aware of possible seizure and how to administer appropriate first aid.

Hearing Impaired
For those clients who are hard of hearing and/or without speech, the client's interpreter may be required to remain in the room during treatment. Always verbally address the client on relevant issues not the interpreter. Look directly at the client when speaking. Do not exaggerate or emphasise words by distorting your mouth, as this will make lip reading more difficult for the client. Write down information as appropriate. Reassure the client and establish a satisfactory means of communication before commencing treatment. e.g. have client agree to you discussing with interpreter.

HIV
Clients with HIV should be treated as any other client. However if on a high dose of medication or in a frail state then the *Reflexology Urgent Care Routine* is most appropriate, with the addition of treatment to the thymus, spleen, adrenals, liver and lymphatics. Pressure should be lighter than might be considered appropriate for the foot size. (See page 92)

Clients suffering from Mental Disorders
Mental Health covers a very wide field. Here the intent is to bring to mind self and patient care when dealing with the more serious diagnosed conditions, especially when instability is an issue.

Consideration should be the same as for elderly and disabled clients. In addition be very reassuring. Give explanations to guardian/ carer/parent if appropriate. If instability is an issue take safety precautions. Ensure others know where you are. Ensure you have a clear escape route. Treat only when under the appropriate supervision of a health care professional. Be aware that some situations may render treatment contra-indicated at a particular time and unless you feel your training has been such as to cover dealing with special and more serious mental disorders, then these clients may be contra-indicated for your treatment. To optimise support for the patient/client C.P.D. (continuing professional development) would be advantageous.

Pregnancy

While reflexology in pregnancy has proven to be rewarding and beneficial in relation to specific symptoms, only those therapists who have undertaken specific training in the understanding of the various aspects of natural physiological changes and the abnormal changes that can occur during pregnancy and labour should offer treatment or self help advice. Either specialised training of at least 20 hours within the normal training course or C.P.D should be undertaken prior to treatment of a pregnant client. Prospective clients (mothers) should seek a therapist who has undertaken additional specific training in this field.

Visually Impaired

Keep the pathways clear making sure there are no areas where this client could collide or trip. Stay close by and guide continuously if necessary. Explain your intention before starting treatment. Give written copies of all documentation, but not necessarily the completed consultation sheet – just a sample of the one you use in the clinic. Explain after-care and offer to give this explanation in writing. Written consent may be difficult. Some clients will be able to make a signature. Some will have a carer to sign on their behalf or to guide them.

Wheelchair-Bound Clients

Be patient and be prepared to treat according to needs. All issues relevant to elderly clients and to those with disabilities should be considered alongside the following:

- Brakes should be on before commencing treatment.
- In the interest of therapist and heath and safety it may be necessary to alter position or remove foot plates, in order to avoid accidental injury to legs/feet or to therapist.
- Ensure the client's knees and legs are supported.
- If client suffers leg muscle spasm, avoid cold wipes and adapt the working position to accommodate.
- Be aware that clients who are immobile tend to feel colder than those who are normally active.
- Address the client always, not the chaperone, on all relevant matters unless this is not appropriate.

Cultural Factors

As with all clients, dignity should be preserved and specific treatment needs should be accommodated. However different needs may include for example a same gender practitioner or only exposing a minimum area of skin. With the latter, therapists may have to adapt their technique. Diversity should be acknowledged and given due respect. Race, colour, creed, religion and gender should form no barrier or exclusion from treatment, but instead the therapist should welcome the opportunity to learn from and share in the knowledge and experience of all those who seek treatment.

Client Aftercare

Ensure the client or their carer understands everything. Where possible give the information in writing. The client will feel good to have the information for reading and digesting later. This can help to reduce worry and possible embarrassment if a client's memory is not too good.

Note

Your own health and safety are important when using adapted techniques if a client cannot weight-bear. Unless you are trained to lift correctly and feel confident and able to do so at the time in question, **DO NOT LIFT!**

PROFESSIONAL THERAPISTS
KNOW YOUR RESPONSIBILITIES

If you take it upon yourself to tell your client/patient the precise organs/glands you are working on, then you should be prepared to take the consequences of your action. If you choose to give this information you should aim to support the reasoning by relating to the information given by the client during the consultation. For example, a reaction found on the ear reflex may correspond to a recent cold.

Many clients/patients who seem calm, logical and sensible while in your company can be caused great anxiety when alone, thinking about your treatment and comments. Few people fully understand the principles of Reflexology and the imagination is a powerful tool. You should always be professional and ethical in your regard to areas or organs being worked on.

Should you feel that the client being treated would benefit from seeking medical advice, or that he/she should be referred to a therapist with different or more appropriate skills, then you are both morally and ethically bound to give this advice to your client.

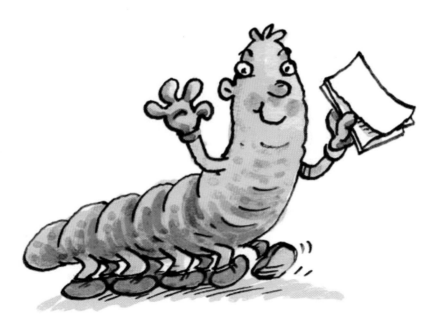

REMEMBER THE S.O.A.P!

Client Documentation and Professional Records
Client records are legal documents and can be subpoenaed in insurance/legal cases. Always follow the guidelines of your professional organisation.

- Do not use the words 'Patient' or 'Cure'
- Use anatomical names in relation to areas where a reaction is felt and to be recorded (i.e. pituitary S = pituitary sensitive). You could add a figure to denote the level of sensitivity, e.g. 1-10 with 10 being the most severe. Use terminology that can be clearly understood.
- Supporting diagrams (in colour if preferred) are fine but totally inadequate on their own merit.

The S.O.A.P method of recording information is well-tried, tested and respected.

S = Subjective Assessment (examination)
This is the client's medical history and lifestyle; the client's perception of his/her condition and what the client says about their complaint.

O = Objective Assessment (examination)
Your notes on visual observations and results from touch. Visual observation is your impression as the client entered your room. Did the client limp? Did they look hunched over? Shoulders raised around ears? Hand clutching leg? Was the client sprightly and full of enthusiasm? What was their facial expression like? What was the FEELING, i.e. palpation of tissue. Were there points of tenderness and/or sensitivity? Take note of temperature, texture, tension, hard skin, lumps, bumps, fluid, suppleness, etc.

A = Assessment on findings
Objective and subjective. The therapist will reach a conclusion and make an assessment of how to proceed.

P = Plan
What the therapist aims to do. The plan of action. To consider a full reflexology routine, symptomatic routine, zone walking. What is the pressure you have decided on? Will there be a referral?

110

CLIENT ARRIVAL TO DEPARTURE

■ Welcome with a smile.

■ Introduce yourself.

■ Take their coat and hang it up.

■ Show client where to sit.

■ Sit close to client, but no closer than 25 inches (63.5cm)

■ Do not sit behind the desk/table but alongside.

■ Inquire if first treatment.

■ Ask reason for visit.

■ Explain what you intend to do and what reflexology is.

■ Complete the consultation and reassure regarding confidentiality.

■ Date the form and then you both sign it (explain why).

■ Ask client if they would like to go to the toilet (show them where it is).

■ Advise client exactly what to take off (shoes, socks/tights). Guide the client onto the couch/chair.

■ Check comfort.

■ Wash your hands in the client's presence or explain you are about to wash your hands.

■ Wipe both feet. Use a separate wipe for each foot.

■ Make a detailed visual examination of each foot.

■ Use Massage/Relaxation techniques on both feet.

- Wrap one foot.

- Treat the other foot (more common to treat right foot first).

- Once the breast reflex is treated change to other foot and treat that.

- Do boost treatment on left foot and then right foot.

- Treat the colon.

- Return to any areas that need further treatment.

- Treat the diaphragm.

- Treat the Solar Plexus.

- Massage/relaxation techniques to both feet

- Wash your hands.

- Give client a small glass of cold water to drink.

- Help client off the couch/chair.

- Offer help with dressing if needed.

- Give after care advice.

- Make a further appointment (if relevant).

- Escort the client to the door/reception.

- Complete the client record sheet.

- File client's notes.

- Clean away ready for next client.

- Prepare the couch/chair with clean towels and tissue.

- Put a clean tissue or mat by the couch/chair for client's feet.

- Check the toilet is clean and all necessities are in place.

- Wash your hands. Drink a fresh juice or some water.

- Have an energy break.

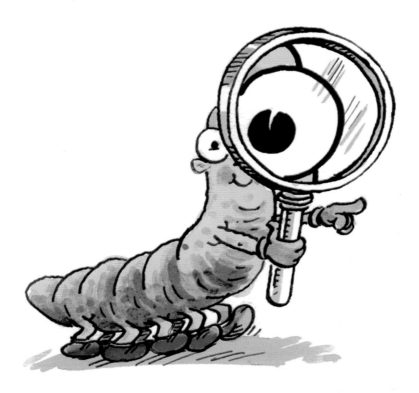

A TYPICAL CONSULTATION FORM

THERAPIST'S NAME

Client Name Address Telephone Number Date of Birth Weight Height Occupation Referred by Reason for Visit Tel. No. Next of Kin (Relationship)	Name of Doctor Address Tel. No.

KNOWN MEDICAL HISTORY

Medication
Previous Illnesses
Family Illnesses
Previous Operations
Accidents/Injuries
Back Problems
Allergies Self/Family
Menstrual Problems (F)
Skin Type
State of Health General

LIFESTYLE

No. of Children
Ages of Children
Marital Status
Smoking (amount)
Drinking (amount)
Balanced Diet
Eating Habits
Regular Exercise
Work Routine
Sleep Pattern
Stress Prone - effects of -
Depression Prone - effects of -

OTHER

Pregnant
Physical Difficulties
Eyesight/Hearing
Posture
Any other condition, disorder or disease you would like to discuss:
Are you receiving other forms of therapy?
When?   Outcomes?
Last visit to GP
Reason   Outcome
Last visit to Hospital
Reason   Outcome

CLIENT'S SIGNATURE: **THERAPIST'S SIGNATURE:**

WHY DO A CONSULTATION SHEET?

Why is there a need for signatures?

Through question and answer the therapist is able to ascertain if the client is suffering with any contra-indications and also it allows the therapist to note areas when caution should be exercised. It is at this time the needs, wants and expectations of the client are established and the therapist can explain the benefits and limitations of the therapy. A consultation helps to build a rapport with the client and builds a picture of the client's health and lifestyle. It gives the client time to talk in a relaxed non-threatening environment and the therapist time to exercise good listening skills.

It is during the consultation that the therapist is able to reassure the client that all information shared with the therapist is completely confidential. To support this the therapist could explain where and how the information is stored (in the UK, storage of information should meet with the requirements of the Data Protection Act).

Asking the Questions

The therapist should ask the questions, listen to the answers, probe for more in-depth information if necessary and then record the outcomes. There is a lot that can be learned from the way the client answers a question and this can be used as a valuable tool in the overall assessment. Yet this is something that is often missed when the client is given the form to complete themselves.

Form Filling

Some people have a 'form phobia' and to be given one to complete in your clinic may cause further stress. Some will not understand the jargon/terminology and will find it easier to write 'No' or become very embarrassed at the thought of having to ask you to explain (even when they have been assured it is alright to do so). Some can neither read nor write though they may first appear capable and verbally articulate. Once you have recorded all the information, go through questions again with the client, confirming you understood their answer and be willing to explain or re-phrase anything that seems unclear to the client. This is an important aspect of consultation and need only take a few minutes (use phrases to affirm clients original response rather than repeat entire question). Give the client the form to read. Allow them a few minutes to do this. New information related to health and lifestyle changes should be recorded at the appropriate session.

Signatures

Next ask for the client's signature, then you should also sign the form in the client's presence and date it.

The client is signing in agreement with the information recorded on the consultation form and in consent to your giving them treatment. You, the therapist, are signing in agreement to the information being kept confidential, apart from notifiable diseases that must be reported by law; or in a case where the client is a serious danger to themselves or someone else, or in the case of a minor in danger.

Note

Relevant information in relation to health previously omitted by the client either through memory lapse or for personal reasons should be recorded and dated at the appropriate session and the client's signature obtained.

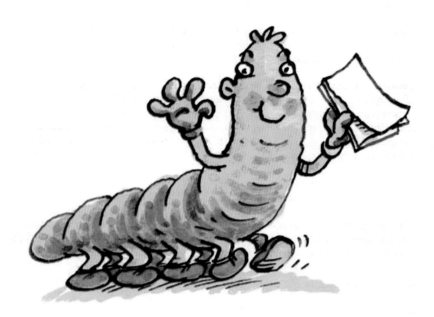

WHY A TREATMENT RECORD SHEET?

WHY A CASE HISTORY?

The treatment record sheet gives the therapist an opportunity to record reactions and outcomes accurately, allowing him/her to build a quick reference system as well as complete a visual picture of the client's progress. All therapists are legally required to keep accurate records. These can be called for in the case of a dispute, especially by a court of law. Clients are also entitled to see/read their records and may also ask for a copy (these procedures are covered by the Data Protection Act in the UK). Keeping accurate records forms part of the contract for membership with a professional organisation and with the therapist's insurance company.

A treatment record sheet should be completed after each treatment and a case history summary completed at the end of a course of treatments. Many therapists like to support their written notes with a coloured diagram of the areas of reaction. This can be very helpful, particularly for students seeking clarification from their tutor and for therapists under supervision. However, this method of recording is not adequate as a stand alone record. Accurately maintained records may be used for research purposes.

CASE HISTORY SUMMARY/EVALUATION

While all therapists are expected to keep detailed notes, students are expected to keep detailed notes on history and evaluation. In writing the case history notes you might consider the following:

■ Review each treatment and final outcome

■ Draw a conclusion based on that review

■ You could note in the final analysis the client's involvement and opinion and your own understanding and feelings about the sessions individually and/or in general.

■ You might like to draw an analogy with similar cases you have treated.

■ Does your lack of experience have a bearing on the outcome?

- Does your experience have a bearing on the outcome?

- In conclusion your notes must show reasoned for argument in relation to outcomes.

SAMPLE TREATMENT RECORD SHEET

Reactions since last treatment Sleeping much better					
Date/ Time	**Right Foot**	**Left Foot**	**Client Comments**	**Therapist's Comments**	**Therapist's Signature**
15.03.04	Sinuses C	Sinuses S	Very Sensitive	Did not seem to relax	C. Pillar
Home Care Advice given No stimulants for at least six hours (i.e. coffee)					

IS IT NECESSARY TO GIVE A BOWL OF WATER?

IS IT NECESSARY TO USE OILS AND CREAMS?

Reflexology is a treatment always performed on clean feet. Offensive odour may cause embarrassment to both therapist and client alike. The client will not relax and enjoy a treatment if they feel that you, the therapist, are being subjected to unpleasant smells or excessively sweaty feet.

It is a good idea to offer a bowl of water to those clients/patients who have not had a chance to take a shower or bath for some time. A building worker, for example, who has been in his shoes and socks all day is likely to sweat more than the average housewife. The water used should not contain chemical additives or perfume but 5ml of *pre-blended* Aromatherapy Oil (e.g. lavender at 1%) or some salt or cider vinegar is acceptable just to refresh. The water must not be hot as this will heat the feet artificially and as a result circulation will be increased. Further Reflexology may over stimulate and result in the treatment being less effective than it might otherwise be.

For those clients/patients who do not need a bowl of water the feet can be refreshed by wiping with a pad soaked in a refreshing solution, e.g. tonic, witch hazel or surgical spirit or a pre-prepared antiseptic tissue wipe.

It is important to give a Reflexology Treatment on dry feet or hands. This gives the opportunity to feel and work deeply without the hands sliding over the flesh. If the flesh feels damp I always dry the skin thoroughly after the cleaning or refreshing process. Some therapists like to use an Aromatherapy based cream, especially on dry or problem feet. I can see no reason why this cream cannot be applied at the end of the Reflexology part of the treatment and the final massage performed with it. Should the cream be used for the opening relaxation movements then it must be completely removed prior to the Reflexology treatment.

Note
Aromatherapy based cream should always be blended by a qualified Aromatherapist before being used by a Reflexologist. This cream must be in very low dilution ¼% to ½% maximum.

The therapist is in a position to advise the client/patient of the benefits of bathing the feet daily and of the necessity to change socks or tights at least once a day in order to keep feet fresh and healthy. Do exercise tact and thoughtfulness when giving such advice.

In the case of excessively sweaty feet, the client should be advised to soak their feet as often as possible in a bowl of warm water to which has been added some lemon juice or vinegar. Better still would be to use 5ml (1 teaspoon) of pre-blended Aromatherapy Essential Oil in the bath or foot bowl. These oils should be purchased from a professional Aromatherapist.

Note
Excessively sweaty feet can benefit from regular Reflexology treatments. There are a number of recorded incidents where this problem has been successfully treated.

VISUAL EXAMINATION SHEET

Check and note information in relation to both feet.

CONDITIONS/ ABNORMALITIES	POTENTIAL DISORDERS CURRENT/PAST
Arch High	Hip, knee, lower back; headaches
Arch High	Leg aches; poor circulation in toes/foot
Athlete's Foot	Contagious infection; low immunity
Blood Vessels - Enlarged	Sluggish circulation; under-active reflex
Bunion	Back problems; thyroid disorder
Cold Spot	Imbalance in the reflex area, possibly under-active, low energy levels
Colour Blue	Poor circulation; low oxygen levels in blood; thyroid or respiratory disorder
Colour Red	Blocked energy related to reflex; systemic disorder; inflammation in foot; toxins in blood; poor venous return; increase in size of small blood vessels in the area over active reflex (just hot)
Colour White	Reynaud's syndrome; poor circulation; under-active reflex (just cold)
Colour Yellow	Tends to relate to toxins, smoking, chemicals, drugs, medication
Corns	Low energy in corresponding reflex; pressure/rubbing on the foot
Cracks	Low energy in corresponding reflex; diet low in fat/water; posture problems

121

CONDITIONS/ ABNORMALITIES	POTENTIAL DISORDERS CURRENT/PAST
Dry Skin	Hormone imbalance; thyroid disorder; digestive imbalance; sinusitis; reaction to medication; dehydration; water metabolism disorder
Hammer Toes	Headaches; sinusitis; gum/teeth problems; low energy to related reflex.
Hard Skin	Low energy to reflex; posture problem; back, hip, knee problem
Hot Spots	Over active reflex
Odour Acetone	Low energy in elimination system; diabetes
Odour Cheese	Congested with toxins; low energy to digestive system
Puffiness/Swelling	Low energy in reflex; rheumatoid arthritis; hormonal imbalance; kidney; heart low in energy; diabetes; gravitational cause (e.g. standing for long periods)
Scars	Possible energy blockage in location
Sweat - Oily Feet	Overworked adrenal gland; stress
Sweat - Moist	Thyroid imbalance; overload on nervous system; allergy
Tense/Limp Foot	Reflecting inner feelings; body organs (tense/limp)
Toe Nails	Similar to hammer toes (see above), plus sluggish reflex within the related zone/s; dandruff, hair loss/thinning
Verruca	Low energy to reflex; lowered immune system; infection

Note
Record any other changes to the feet and observe changes during the course of treatment

ABNORMALITIES OF THE FEET THAT AFFECT OTHER REFLEX ZONES

1. Infected toe nails normally indicate that the reflex zones to the head area have been affected. Sugar, alcohol or cigarette use might be high. Migraine could even be a problem.

2. Hammer Toes and similar deformities suggest the head and face zones, which include teeth, gums and sinuses, could have been affected.

3. Flat feet could indicate the reflex zones to the spinal column are affected. There may also be some digestive problems, such as constipation.

4. Congestion in the ankle area could indicate affected reflex zones in the pelvis or hip joint.

5. Bunions/Hallux Vulgus, could suggest possible congestion in the reflex zones of the cervical and thoracic spine, the thyroid or the pancreas.

6. Corns showing anywhere on the feet (whatever the initial cause) indicate that the reflex zone for that area might be affected. If the corn presents itself in the shoulder reflex point or similar area, this would naturally tell us that there might well be a problem in the shoulder area but could also suggest congestion/ energy blockage in the entire zone.

7. Athlete's Foot (*Tinea Pedis*). Observe carefully the spread of the infection, it may cover more than one zone. When there is infection present or there is a change of colour or texture radiating from that area it usually indicates an energy blockage in the affected zone. If Athlete's Foot is present or if there is any doubt, work on the client's corresponding hand but do examine the feet first.

8. I believe that any change in the skeletal, muscular or tissue structure of the foot could, like Athlete's Foot, suggest an energy blockage in the corresponding area of the body. Therefore, even if the client does not complain of problems within an area where we get visible signs of such, it is still worthwhile to work on those areas even if the skin is thick. Eventually we should get results. It would also be helpful to work on the corresponding area of the hand, after you have completed the routine on both feet. (Never break from the foot routine to treat the hand).

THE 7 'T's OF TREATMENT

Temperature
May indicate poor circulation due to a vascular disturbance, it may also indicate that the air temperature is very cold/very hot or the person is inadequately clothed for the weather conditions.

Tenderness
May indicate energy blockages, health disorders, stress.

Tension
May be due to anxiety in general or for the moment, also stress or lack of sleep.

Texture
May indicate dehydration, inadequate dietary requirements, allergies, circulation disorders.

Ticklishness
May be due to stress, tension, shyness, not used to being touched.

Touch
The contact between therapist, hands and client.

Tremors
May be due to neurological disorder, nervousness, stress.

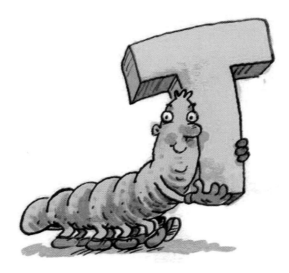

HANDS

While this book makes reference to treatment of the hands, there is insufficient space here to include all the information on how to give a full treatment to the hands. I have, however, included a diagram of the hand which will enable you to have a visual reference of the relevant reflexes.

A good knowledge of hand reflexology is a very valuable tool for self help reflexology treatment and also for the professional therapist who may find themselves in the situation where it is not possible, for a variety of reasons, to treat the feet. My book on hand reflexology is very explicit on how to do the movements and it takes the reader through the sequence of a full treatment on the hand as well as giving the information on how to treat reflexes specific to a particular condition.

RIGHT HAND
DORSUM

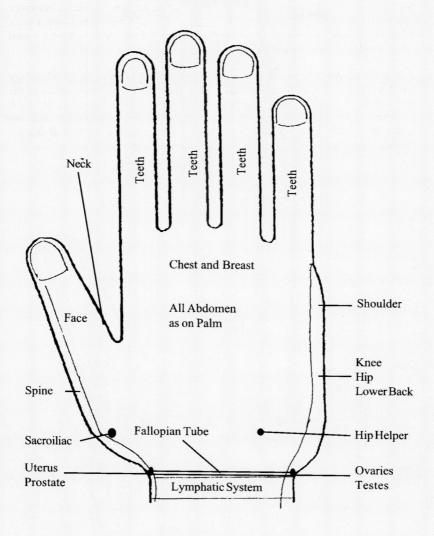

Neck

Teeth

Teeth

Teeth

Teeth

Chest and Breast

All Abdomen
as on Palm

Shoulder

Face

Knee
Hip
Lower Back

Spine

Sacroiliac

Fallopian Tube

Hip Helper

Uterus
Prostate

Lymphatic System

Ovaries
Testes

6) **Dorsum Squeeze**
Stretch your fingers across the dorsum. Thumbs on sole of foot. Squeeze and release twice. Move down the foot working in this manner (take care that you do not pinch loose skin).

7) **Sole Stretch**
Cup the heel of one foot in your hand. Place the other hand with the palm on the ball of the foot and the fingers resting on the toes. Use this top hand to push the foot away from you and hold to a slow count of three. Next wrap your fingers (nearest to toes) around the dorsum and gently pull the foot towards you (not the toes). Hold to a slow count of three (omit or do very gently if any foot problems or arthritis present).

8) **Spine Twist**
Put both hands alongside each other on the inside of the foot (medial edge) thumbs on the sole, fingers across the dorsum (top). This will mean that the edge of the foot is trapped in the webbing between your index finger and your thumb. Both index fingers should be touching. Hold the hand near the ankle steady. Use the other hand to twist the foot gently back and forth a couple of times. Next move both hands just a little along the foot towards the toes and repeat the action. Continue in this way until you reach the toes then slide both hands to the ankle and repeat the movement.

1) **Greet the Feet**

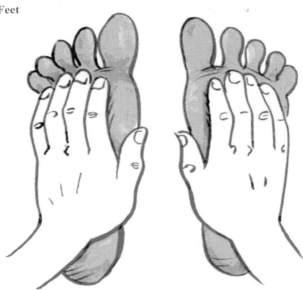

2) **Circulation Boost**

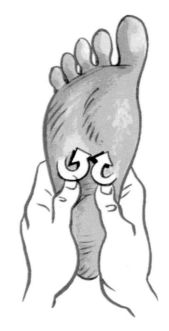

3)   Toe Fan

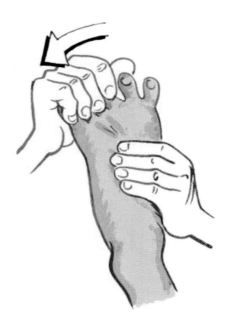

4)   Toe Stretch, Toe Rotation

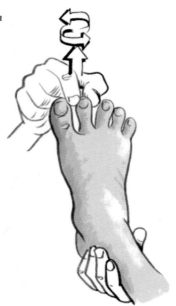

5)   **Metatarsal Kneeding**

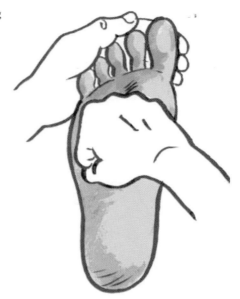

6)   **Dorsum Squeeze**

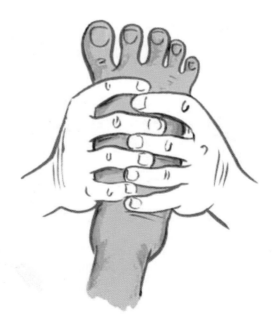

135

7)   **Sole Stretch**

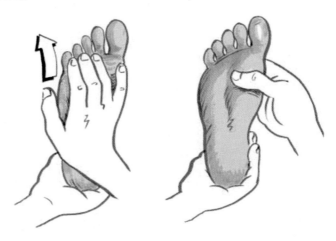

8)   **Spine Twist**

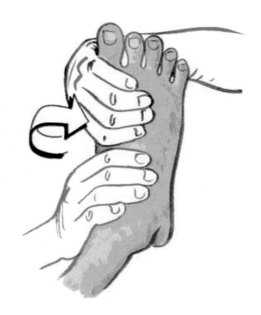

REFLEX MAP

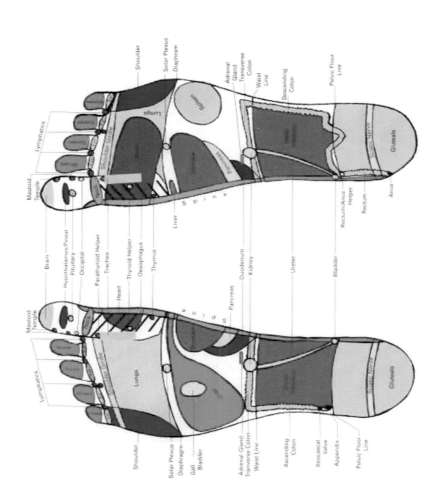

REFLEX MAP

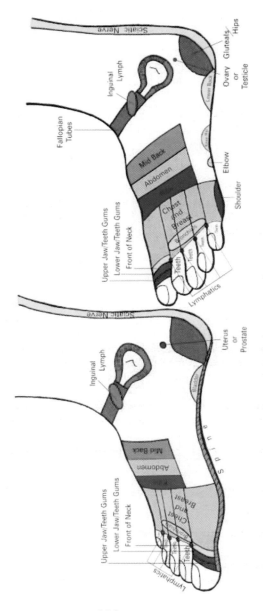

WORKING TIPS
FOR THE THERAPIST

■ Welcome the client with a smile.

■ Conduct a consultation. Re-assure the client about confidentiality.

■ During the consultation ask the questions and listen carefully to the answers. Acknowledge what the client is saying and write down the information.

■ Establish that there are no contra-indications. Make a note of areas of caution.

■ Explain reflexology to the client. Keep it brief. Some people are very interested and will want to know more. In this case, of course, you should explain further, but do not fall into the trap of trying to explain all you know about the therapy.

■ In explaining the therapy, you could talk about mirrored images of the body being reflected onto the foot.

■ In explaining 'energy blockage' to your client you might draw an analogy with a congested road in the location of a large open air concert or football match: the police are working to keep the traffic moving on a road which, under normal circumstances, carries daily traffic without problem. The thumb acts as the police, moving the congestion through the body, making way for the free flow of energy.

■ Use warm towels to wrap the foot and the client in cool weather. Use a blanket to cover the client in cold weather. This is comforting and re-assuring.

■ Protect the client's modesty when moving legs and feet.

■ Keep refreshing antiseptic wipes in a sealed container in the fridge for use in very hot weather.

■ Do not lean on the client when working.

■ The therapist should sit at a comfortable distance from the feet which should not necessitate the arms being fully outstretched.

- It is necessary to use both hands; one to steady, one to work.

- Keep your thumb/finger in contact with the skin.

- When doing your caterpillar walk, take very small bite-sized movements, as though you are walking over a festive orange, covered in cloves. You must make contact with every clove head. Alternatively imagine you are working on an old-fashioned pin cushion where you must make contact with each pin head.

- At some point in our lives most of us have attempted to complete a jigsaw puzzle. Now try to imagine the reflex points on the feet/hands as a piece of a jigsaw puzzle which, when integrated with anatomy and physiology will give you a picture of the client's overall health and well-being.

- Do not raise the working joint/knuckle too high as this will create stress on the joint, resulting in long term discomfort and furthermore your nail will stick into the client.

- Imagine you have an eye in your thumb/finger. Look and feel for changes: cold spots, fluid spots, hot spots, granulations, tension or just a different feel to what you might expect.

- I work with the pad of my thumb/finger. Some therapists use the side/edge of the thumb/finger. I have seen on more than one occasion long term nail damage as a direct result of this technique, although some argue that it is a result of incorrect technique and not the use of the side/edge of the thumb/finger. I am not convinced by this argument.

- My experience dictates that it is not absolutely necessary to work the right foot with the right hand or *vice versa* but it is usually more comfortable for both client and therapist.

- I do not recommend the use of talcum powder for the following reasons: it may cause allergic reaction in susceptible clients and it creates dust, allowing the therapist's lungs to be subjected to a constant source of possible irritation.

- Ideally work with the client's feet or hands at the therapist's chest level.

- Do not lay the client flat, as it is necessary to observe the client's face and this also offers a measure of security for the client.

- A professional treatment couch, one with a lift up back rest and no cross stays at the end is ideal, but make sure it is well-padded on the sitting area, so as to protect the client's coccyx (lower back).

- A padded, professional chair with an electric motor would be even more suitable; however the expense will make this prohibitive in many cases.

- A U-shaped chair may cause congestion in the abdominal area.

- Some reclining chairs may elevate the legs too much, especially in a 40/45 minute treatment. The action of gravity may allow more blood than normal to rush to the brain. Most clients do not practice standing on their heads and therefore being in this position for the duration of treatment can result in the client feeling very unwell.

- Sit on a therapist's stool, one with an adjustable back rest and height adjuster is best. The stool should also have casters as this makes for ease of movement and hand changes and also helps prevent back and shoulder strain (if you are able to move with ease and adjust height).

- For maximum comfort for the client, pad the lower back, under the knees and under the ankles.

- Keep a clean uniform for emergencies (accidental spillages).

- Turn mobile phone ring tones off and ask the client to do the same.

- Ensure that the business phone sounds are out of earshot for the client. These bring back memories of work and home life and can cause stress.

- Do not answer the phone during a treatment or have other interruptions.

- Never divulge to a client that you are alone in a building.

- If you do work alone, have an emergency panic button fitted.

- Always have an escape route planned.

- Mobile therapists should always make sure that someone knows where they are at all times during working hours.

- Do not have strong smells in the clinic as this can be overpowering, disliked by the client and can linger on the clothes. Subtle smells can be pleasing to the senses and linger in the memory.

- Do not smoke in the building or allow the client to smoke.

- Do not drink alcohol in the building or allow the client to do so either.

- Do not play music during the treatment unless you have checked that it is agreeable to the client. If the client is willing to have music, make a note of what you have played, it may be requested on another visit.

- Use fresh flowers sparingly. Some clients may have allergies to them. If you use artificial flower arrangements make sure that they are kept clean and fresh looking.

- If your client takes medication and there is a possibility that this might be needed during the treatment. Ask them to put the container into their shoe. This will prevent the therapist having to search in an emergency and it also helps the client to remember to take it home again.

- Complete the treatment record sheet prior to the next client's session and always record any advice given.

- When giving home care advice , in relation to drinking water, you could suggest an increase in intake if necessary, rather than letting the client drink lots of water. A sudden increase in intake of water might encourage disturbed sleep and numerous trips to the toilet; prompting the question whether it is the reflexology or the water working (this is especially important on the first one or two visits, so that outcomes of the treatment can be more accurately assessed).

- Take a minimum of fifteen minutes break between each client. Six clients a day should be the maximum to ensure the therapist is not overworked and that the clients get a good treatment (value for money).

- You must take care of your own health before trying to care for others. My recommendation – rest, good food, fresh air, exercise and relaxation, blended with regular treatments from another all help to make a good therapist.

THE REFLEXOLOGY TREATMENT

How to Perform A Full Treatment

1. Always commence the treatment with the *right foot* (the 'physical' foot), unless the point you are concentrating on is specifically on the left foot only.

2. Follow points 1 through to 40 on the right foot as illustrated in the sequence on the following pages.

3. Ignore the ones marked specifically for the left foot only. Once you reach number 40 (Breast), go back and start again at number 1 (Diaphragm Line) but this time work on the *left foot* (the 'emotional' foot).

4. Follow points 1 through to 40 on the left foot as illustrated. Ignore the ones marked specifically for the right foot only.

5. Once you reach number 40 continue by following the instructions for both feet, from number 41 to conclusion.

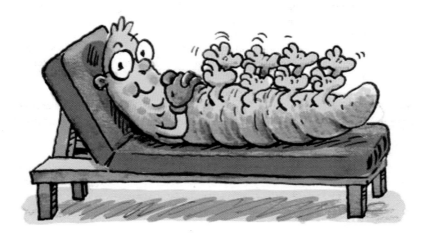

REFLEXOLOGY ROUTINE AND SEQUENCE FOR FULL TREATMENT

1. Diaphragm Line

Location
Zone 1 – Zone 5

Area
Sole across the foot from medial
to lateral side, directly under ball of foot

Digit
Thumb

Technique
Caterpillar Walk

Hold
Either sole support or foot wrap.

Treatment
Place the palmar surface of the thumb on the diaphragm line directly below the ball of the foot. Caterpillar walk across the reflex from Zone 1 to Zone 5.

How Often
3 Walks would be average. However this can be increased to 5 in the stressed client and returned to periodically during the sequence to aid relaxation in the very sensitive.

Note
The diaphragm will also be treated 3 times in the conclusion of the treatment.

DIAPHRAGM LINE

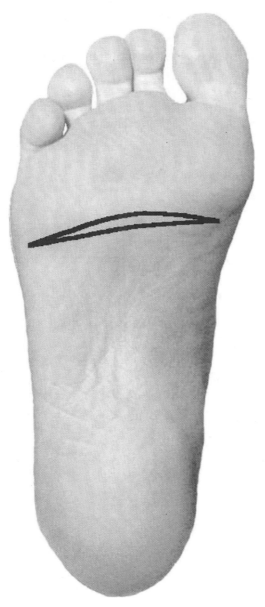

2. Solar Plexus

Location
Zone 2 - Zone 3

Area
Sole, straddling diaphragm line

Digit
Thumb

Technique
Press-in technique or pin point technique

Hold
Either sole support or foot wrap.

Treatment
Place the palmar surface of the distal joint (first joint) of the working thumb so it straddles the diaphragm.
Give three distinct on/off presses into the reflex. Alternatively use pin point technique.

How Often
Do treatment sequence twice at beginning and twice at the end of treatment.

Note
If reflex is very sensitive hold thumb pressure for between ten and fifteen seconds. Work to client's tolerance level. When working on an overall very sensitive foot, return to treat the solar plexus, following treatment of adrenal gland.

SOLAR PLEXUS

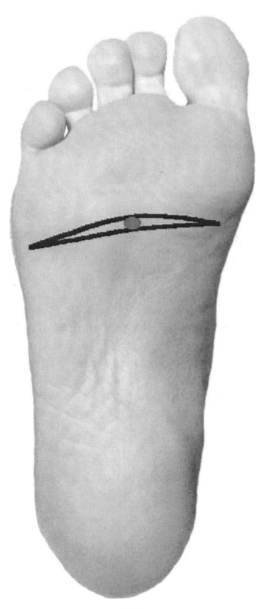

3. Head – Brain - Face

Location
Zone 1 Big Toe

Area
Both sides, top, back and
front of toe

Digit
Thumb – Index Finger

Technique
Caterpillar Walk

Hold
Beak hold, thumb/finger grip, toe bend.

Treatment
Horseshoe shape - up outside edge of toe, over top, down other side.
Work over back of toe from base to top. Work down front of toe to
bottom.

(i)   Use the working thumb to caterpillar walk up the outside of
        the big toe over the top and down the other side. (Head/Brain)

(ii)   Hold the foot in a foot wrap. Use the working thumb to
        caterpillar walk up the back of the toe from the neck of the toe
        to the top of the toe. Use as many movements as necessary to
        cover the area. (Back of Head/Brain).

(iii)   Hold toe in finger and thumb grip. Alternatively use foot wrap.
        Use the index finger to caterpillar walk down the front of the
        toe, from top to neck. (Face).

How often
Do movement twice. If a reactive reflex or a related condition, do
each movement twice more.

Note
As we work the big toe we are not just treating the pituitary, pineal and
hypothalamus but also the sense organs of sight, hearing, smell and
taste, as well as gums and teeth.

HEAD - BRAIN - FACE

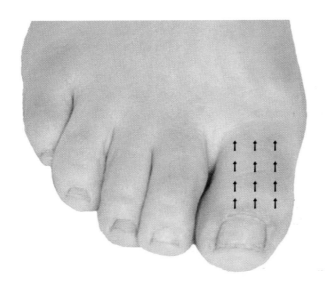

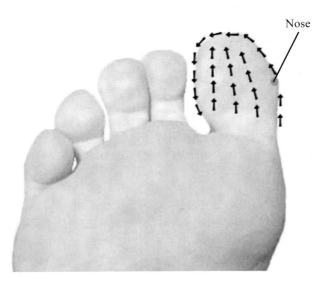

Nose

4. Front of Neck – Back of Neck

Location	*Area*
Zone 1 Big Toe	Neck of big toe – back and front

Digit	*Technique*
Thumb + Index finger	Caterpillar Walk

Hold
Front: Thumb/Finger Grip
Back: Hand Wrap

Treatment
Place the digit on the outer edge of the neck of the big toe, pointing towards the little toe. This position will be the starting point for both front and back of neck. Use finger on front and thumb on the back.

Caterpillar walk across the neck of the toe from outside to inside. Stop between toe one and toe two. Firstly on top, the front of neck, then on the bottom, on the back of the neck.

How Often
Do the treatment three times on each side. If a reactive reflex or a related condition presenting, do the treatment once more.

Note
The base of the toe is very small therefore all the reflexes of the neck are to be found in both the front and back. However experience has proven that certain areas react more favourably on one side than the other.

Front of neck reflex: adenoids, larynx, throat, thyroid, parathyroid, pharynx, tonsils, epiglottis, vocal cords and Eustachian tube.
Back of neck reflex tends to react to energy disturbance relative to that area.

FRONT OF NECK – BACK OF NECK

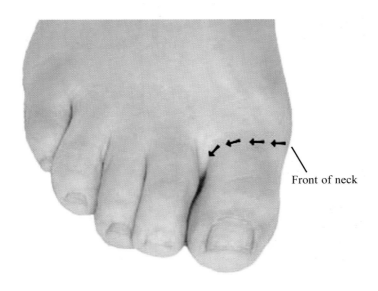

Front of neck

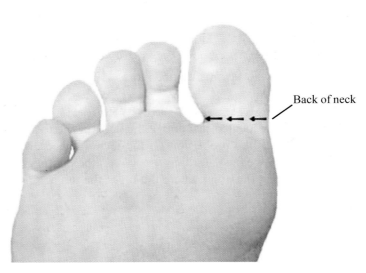

Back of neck

5. Occipital, Mastoid Process, Temple

Location
Zone 1 Big Toe
(side next to toe two)

Area
Big toe base very close to lateral edge

Digit
Thumb

Technique
Caterpillar Walk (bites) and Thumb Presses

Hold
Foot Wrap.

Treatment
Place the thumb with tip pointing upwards on the base of the big toe. Caterpillar walk up the toe for three bites, from neck of toe (usually arriving just below the slight protrusion). Stop at this point and give three distinct on/off presses on the occipital reflex. Caterpillar walk one further bite up the toe. Stop on this mastoid reflex and give three on/off presses on the reflex. Caterpillar walk a further two bites up the toe. Stop on the temple reflex (narrowest part of toe) and give three distinct on/off presses on the reflex.

How Often
Do the treatment once. If a reactive reflex or a related condition presenting, do the treatment once more.

Note
Occipital reflex located just above the neck of the toe and just under the natural ball like protrusion on the lateral aspect. Mastoid reflex located just above the natural protrusion on the lateral aspect. Temple reflex located at the point where the tip of the toe begins to narrow.

OCCIPITAL, MASTOID PROCESS, TEMPLE

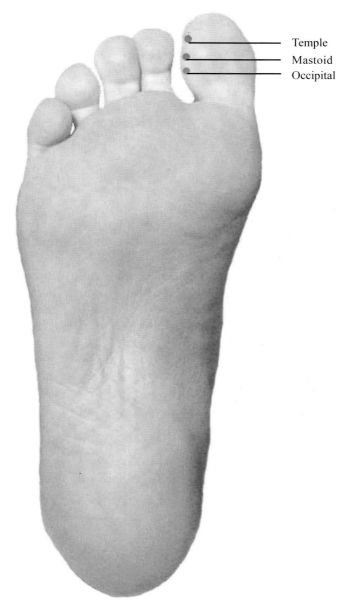

Temple

Mastoid

Occipital

6.   Pituitary – Pineal Gland, Hypothalamus

Location
Zone 1 Big Toe

Area
Centre of widest point on the pad of
the big toe

Digit
Thumb

Technique
Thumb press, Pressure Circles.

Hold
Thumb/Finger support

Treatment
Put your thumb on the widest part of the pad of the big toe, thumb tip
pointing towards the tip of the toe. Give three distinct pressure circles/
rotations on the pituitary gland.
Move one tiny point up the toe towards the tip. Turn your thumb onto
its outer edge (this will correspond with the outer edge of the toe)
make three distinct pressure circles on the hypothalamus. Turn your
thumb onto the opposite edge (closest to fingers). Make three distinct
Pressure Circles on the pineal gland. All three reflexes are in very
close proximity

How often
Do treatment once. If a reactive reflex or a related condition presenting,
do the movements twice more.

Note
When treating pituitary gland: the working thumb can come in from the
top of the toe to locate the reflex, then the hook in and back up technique
can be used.

PITUITARY - PINEAL GLAND, HYPOTHALAMUS

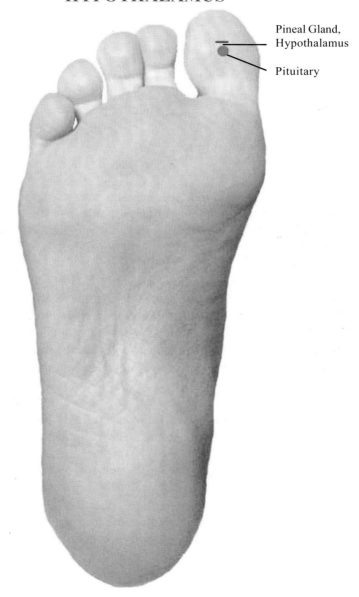

Pineal Gland,
Hypothalamus

Pituitary

7. Sinuses/Cranial Nerves

Location
Zone 2-5
Four small toes

Area
Sides-top-back of toes

Digit
Index finger – Thumb

Technique
Caterpillar Walk – Push/Roll

Hold
Both beak hold and toe bend

Treatment
Use the index finger to treat the cranial nerves. Begin in between big toe and toe two. Caterpillar walk up the side, over the top and down the other side (of toe two) in a horseshoe shape. Repeat the movement on the remaining three toes.

Next use the thumb to caterpillar walk up the back of each toe, beginning with toe two. Then caterpillar walk up each toe to the bulb (fat part). As the tip of the thumb reaches the bulb, use a push-slide type movement on the bulb. This part of the movement will use a deeper pressure and act as if pushing the bulb upwards to roll over the top of the toe (may be sensitive in those who suffer nasal or general allergy type problems).

How often
Do treatment twice. If a reactive reflex or a related condition presenting, repeat the movements. For chronic sinusitis do the movements a total of four times.

Note
A reaction directly under the bulb of either toe two or toe three can relate to the eye and under the bulb of toe four or toe five can relate to ears. However due to nerve proximity toe 3 tends to react for either.

SINUSES/CRANIAL NERVES

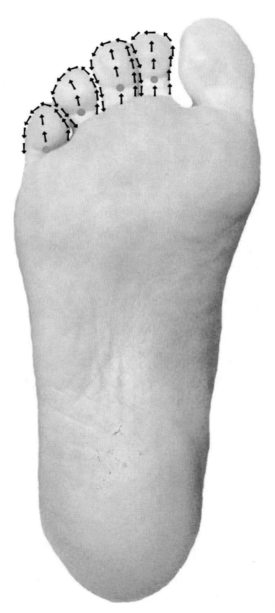

8. Teeth – Gums – Face – Jaw

Location
Zone 1 – Zone 5

Area
Dorsum all five toes

Digit
Index Finger

Technique
Caterpillar Walk

Hold
Thumb finger grip or sole support

Treatment
Place the index finger on the top of the big toe nail, tip of finger pointing towards the leg. Caterpillar walk down the big toe, from top to base. Use as many movements as necessary in order to treat the width of the toe. Next treat remaining four toes in exactly the same way.

How Often
Do the movement twice on each toe. For a reactive reflex or a related condition, do the treatment once more.

Note
All teeth and the gums are treated on the big toe in general. Hence the big toe is also treated in this sequence.

Incisors and Canine teeth	-	Toe two
Premolars	-	Toe three
Molars	-	Toe four
Wisdom	-	Toe five

A reaction on to toe 3 might also relate to inner ear.

TEETH – GUMS – FACE – JAW

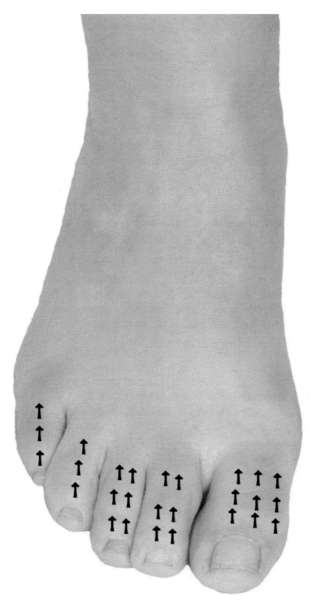

9. Lymphatics of Head - Neck - Thorax

Location
Zone 1 – Zone 5

Area
Webbing between toes

Digit
Thumb and Index Finger

Technique
Pinch, twist – pressure circles

Hold
Finger wrap

Treatment
Very gently pinch the webbing between the toes. Start between the big toe and toe two, then while holding the pinch make a slight twist movement. This action will resemble that of clicking your fingers. Now treat the webbing between the remaining toes.

Next use your index finger to caterpillar walk down the top of the foot to the diaphragm area on the thoracic lymphatic reflex.

(i)   Work in the channel/groove located in line with toe one and toe two.

(ii)   Then work down the same channel/groove again but instead of doing the caterpillar walk, do a series of pressure circles.

How Often
Once on each reflex. If a reactive reflex or a related condition presenting, do the movements twice more.

LYMPHATICS OF HEAD - NECK - THORAX

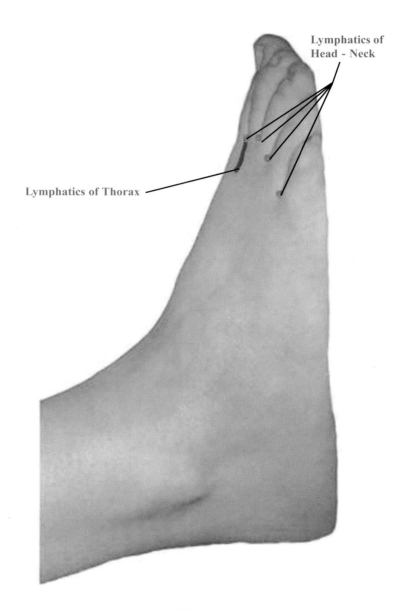

Lymphatics of
Head - Neck

Lymphatics of Thorax

10. Eyes and Ears

Location
Zone 2-3 (Eyes)
Zone 4-5 (Ears)

Area
Ridge at base of toes
(Also related reflex just under bulb)

Digit
Thumb

Technique
Caterpillar Walk

Hold
Foot Wrap.

Treatment
Use the thumb in the caterpillar walk, exerting downward pressure while at the same time allowing the lateral aspect of the thumb to rub along the base of the toes. With toes held back, caterpillar walk along the top of the ridge from toe two to toe five.

How often
Do the movement twice. If a reactive reflex or a related condition presenting, do the movement twice more on the relative reflex.

Note
Eyes between zones 2-3, ears between zones 4-5. Reactions may be felt at the base of the toes when the energy to the reflex is weak. Release the backward toe hold just a little and then make a distinct on-off press into the reflex either on ridge between zones 2-3, or on the ridge between zones 4-5, depending on the area of reaction. Hold each pressure on for about three seconds. Eye-ear related reflex also treated during the treatment of sinuses and cranial nerves.

EYES AND EARS

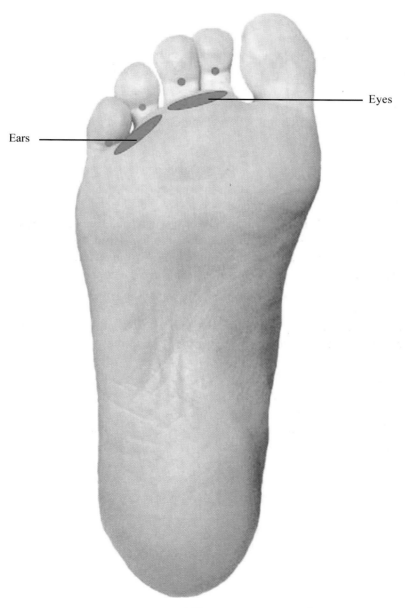

Eyes

Ears

11. Eustachian Tube/Auditory Canal

Location
Between Zones 3-4

Area
Base of toes, dorsum. Ridge on sole at base of toes.

Digit
Index Finger and Thumb

Technique
Pinch – Hold and Push

Hold
Foot Wrap

Treatment
Use index finger on dorsum, in line between toe three and toe four, at the base of the toes, pointing towards the leg. Hold thumb in similar position on sole, pointing toward the heel. Grip the fleshy area not the web. Hold firmly and push towards heel. Keep the hold for three seconds.

How Often
Do the movement once unless ear, nose, throat problems exist when the movement would be done a further three times.

EUSTACHIAN TUBE/AUDITORY CANAL

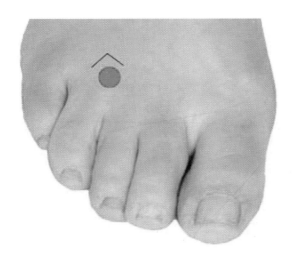

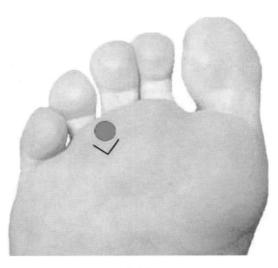

12. Balance

Location
Zone 3 - 4

Area
Base of toe four (Dorsum)

Digit
Index Finger

Technique
Pressure

Hold
Finger and thumb grip.

Treatment
Place index finger on the base/knuckle of toe four (on the dorsum of the foot), tip pointing towards the medial edge of the foot. Give two distinct on-off presses on the reflex.

How Often
Just twice. If reactive reflex or a related condition presenting, do the movement twice more.

Note
If a problem exists and no reaction occurs move the finger and press into the corresponding area on toe three.

BALANCE

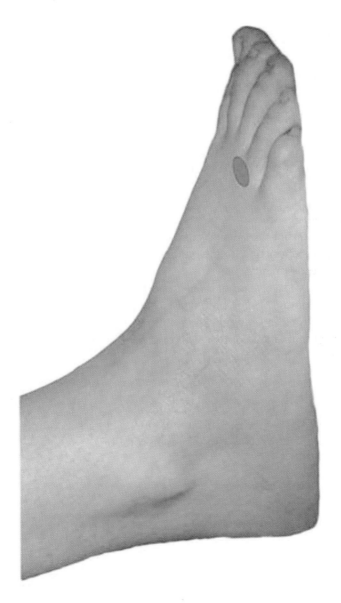

13. Shoulder/Axillary Lymphatics

Location
Between Zones 4-5

Area
Knuckle/Joint on ball of foot
(Metatarsophalangeal joint)

Digit
Thumb and Index Finger

Technique
1) Squeeze
2) Squeeze and Rotate

Hold
Foot Wrap

Treatment
Coming in from the outside edge of the foot, place the index finger on the top of the foot and thumb on the sole. This will be the work position for both movements.
1)   Give two distinct pinch squeezes on the reflex
2)   Continue pinch hold while rotating both digits in a clockwise direction – fingers and thumb should not slide over flesh but should be held in position. The action should mimic that of shoulder rotation.

How Often
If a reactive reflex or related condition presenting, give three further rotations. Then once the full treatment sequence is completed, return to the reflex and give a further seven rotations.

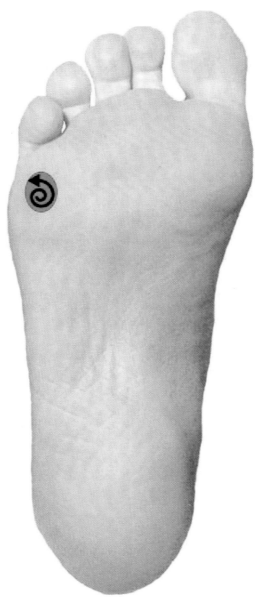

14. Thyroid/Parathyroid (Helper Reflex)

Location
Zone 1 Sole

Area
Along diaphragm line and on ball of foot in line with big toe and toe two

Digit
Thumb

Technique
Caterpillar Walk

Hold
Foot Wrap.

Treatment
Caterpillar walk across diaphragm line, from medial edge of foot. When in line with big toe and toe two, turn your thumb to caterpillar walk up the crease line to the base of the toes.

How Often
Do movement twice. If a reactive reflex or a related condition presenting, do the treatment twice more.

THYROID/PARATHYROID (HELPER REFLEX)

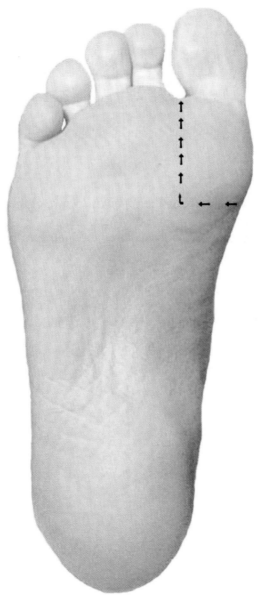

15. Thyroid

Location
Zone 1 ball of foot

Area
Centre of pad, ball of foot

Digit
Thumb

Technique
Pressure Circles (Rotations)

Hold
Foot Wrap.

Treatment
Place the pad of the working thumb on the centre of the pad in the ball of the foot.
Use the working thumb to make three distinct deep pressure circles (rotations) on the reflex

How Often
Once. If a reactive reflex or a related condition presenting, do the treatment twice more (total of nine pressure circles).

THYROID

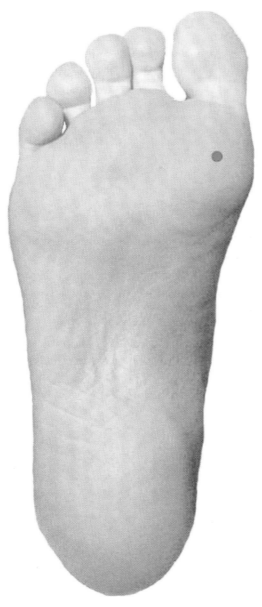

16. Parathyroid

Location
Zone 1

Area
As for number 15 Thyroid, then one point up towards toes and one point over towards toe two.

Digit
Thumb

Technique
Pressure Circles (Rotations)

Hold
Foot Wrap.

Treatment
Place the thumb on the thyroid reflex number 15. Move one point up towards toes and one point over towards toe two.
Use the working thumb to make three distinct deep pressure circles (rotations).

How Often
Once. If a reactive reflex or a related condition presenting, do the treatment twice more (total of nine pressure circles).

PARATHYROID

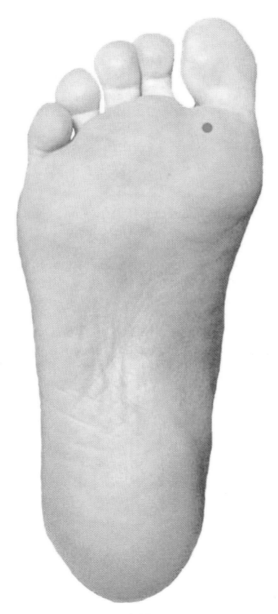

17. Thymus

Location
Zone 1

Area
Ball of foot

Digit
Thumb

Technique
Pressure Circles (Rotations)

Hold
Foot Wrap.

Treatment
Place the thumb on thyroid reflex 15. Move one point down towards the heel and one point towards medial edge of the foot (as close to edge as possible).
Use the working thumb to make three distinct, deep pressure circles (rotations) on the reflex.

How Often
Once. If a reactive reflex or a related condition presenting, do the treatment twice more (total of nine pressure circles).

THYMUS

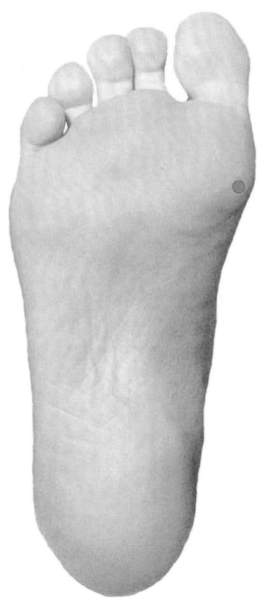

18. Oesophagus – Trachea – Bronchial – Lungs – Shoulder

Location
Zone 1-5

Area
Ball of foot

Digit
Thumb

Technique
Caterpillar Walk

Hold
Foot Wrap

Treatment
From diaphragm to base of all toes.

i)   Caterpillar walk up ball of foot, from diaphragm to base of big toe. This area treats oesophagus for two thirds, final one third towards toe two treats trachea.

ii)   Continue to caterpillar walk up the foot between diaphragm and base of each toe, two, three and four. This movement treats the lungs.

iii)   Continue to caterpillar walk from diaphragm to base of toe five. This movement treats the shoulder area.

How Often
Do movement twice. If a reactive reflex or a related condition presenting, do the treatment twice more.

Note
See diagram for hiatus related reflex. Reaction does not necessarily qualify that a hernia exists. Also note that the bronchial tubes branch from the trachea into the respective lungs.

OESOPHAGUS – TRACHEA – BRONCHIAL – LUNGS – SHOULDER

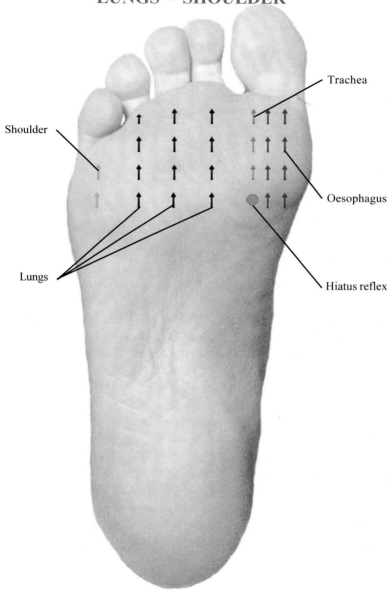

Trachea

Shoulder

Lungs

Oesophagus

Hiatus reflex

19. Chest – Ribs – Lymphatics – Lungs - Shoulders

Location
Zone 2-5

Area
Dorsum of foot, between base of the toes and the area corresponding to the diaphragm line

Digit
Index Finger

Technique
Caterpillar Walk

Hold
Sole Support

Treatment
Place the index finger at the base of toe two (on the dorsum), pointing down the foot, towards the leg.
Caterpillar walk down the foot from the base of each toe to the area corresponding to the diaphragm line. Slide back to the start point each time. Begin with toe two and finish at toe five. Toe two to toe four corresponds to muscles and bones of the chest and also to the general lymphatics of the area as well as the lungs. Toe five corresponds to shoulder.

How Often
Do movement twice. If a reactive reflex or a related condition presenting, do the treatment twice more.

Note
Bony prominence corresponds to the ribs and can be included in treatment. In other words, treat whole area, not just in the grooves. The channels between the metatarsals may be referred to as 'lymphatic valleys'. Main lymphatics between toe 1 and toe 2.

CHEST – RIBS – LYMPHATICS – LUNGS - SHOULDERS

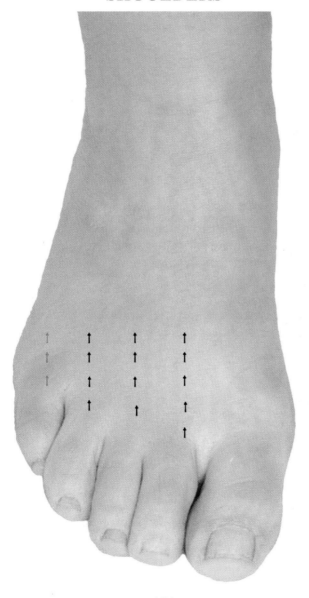

20. Shoulder Girdle – Scapula - Clavicle

Location
Zone 2-5

Area
Sole of foot on the ball. Locate ridge under toes, then move one point down the foot towards the heel.

Digit
Thumb

Technique
Caterpillar Walk

Hold
Foot Wrap.

Treatment
Across the foot from toe two to toe five.
Use the working thumb to caterpillar walk across the foot, just under the ridge, in line with toe two. Finish move in line with toe five.

How Often
Do movement twice. If a reactive reflex or a related condition presenting, do the treatment twice more (again).

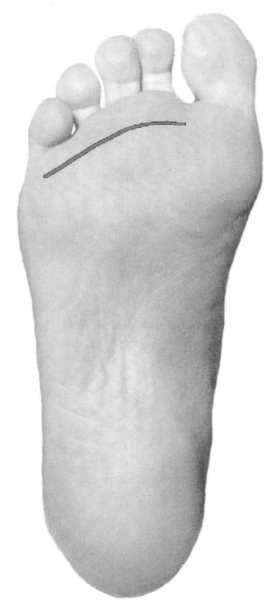

21. Upper Abdomen

Location
Zone 1-5 Sole

Area
Between diaphragm and waist line

Digit
Thumb

Technique
Caterpillar Walk

Hold
Foot Wrap

Treatment
Across the area between diaphragm and waist.
Use the thumb of the working hand to caterpillar walk across the foot from Zone 1 to Zone 5. Do as many movements as necessary to treat the whole area. Then treat the whole area again but this time caterpillar walk across the foot from Zone 5 to Zone 1.

How Often
Do entire movement once in each direction. If a reactive reflex or a related condition presenting, do the treatment once more in each direction.

Note
Location:
Pyloric Sphincter (valve between stomach and duodenum).
Cardia Sphincter (valve between oesophagus and stomach)

Cardia Sphincter tends to be more reactive on the right foot.

UPPER ABDOMEN

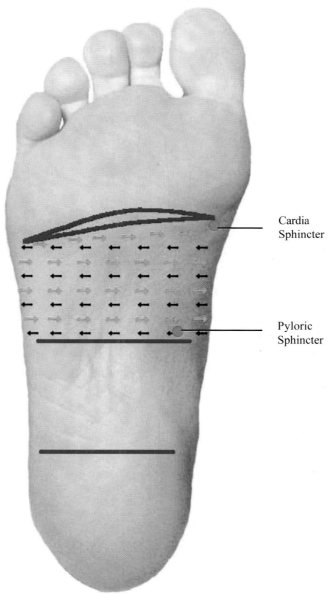

Cardia
Sphincter

Pyloric
Sphincter

22. Gall Bladder – RIGHT FOOT ONLY

Location
Between Zone 3 and
Zone 4

Area
Upper Abdomen

Digit
Thumb

Technique
Pressure

Hold
Foot Wrap.

Treatment
Place the thumb on upper abdomen in line with gap between toes 3-4.
With the tip of the thumb touching the diaphragm line, use the entire
first joint (distal joint) to give two deep presses into the reflex.

How Often
Do two presses only. If a reactive reflex or a related condition presenting,
do the treatment twice more (total 6 presses).

Note
If gall stones present, start with a light pressure, gradually increasing to
client's tolerance level.

GALL BLADDER – RIGHT FOOT ONLY

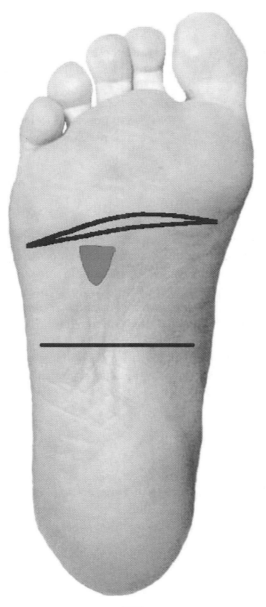

22. Cardiac/Heart Reflex - LEFT FOOT ONLY

Location
Zone 4 – Zone 1

Area
Specific reflex on left foot only. Sole and top of foot between the base of the toes and the diaphragm.

Digit
Sole - Thumb
Top - Index Finger

Technique
Small pressure circles (rotations)
Large pressure circles (rotations)

Hold
Toe Bend

Treatment
i)   Begin with the working thumb resting across the sole on the ball of the foot, just above the diaphragm, in line with toe 3 and toe 4.Give two deep pressure circles/rotations on the spot.
ii)   Put the index finger on the corresponding point on the top of the foot and again give two deep pressure circles/rotations.
iii)   Next move the index finger in 7 distinct large circles covering the area from toe 4 to toe 1, between diaphragm and toes.
iv)   Use your thumb to repeat the 7 large circles on the ball of the foot (sole).

How Often
Do the movement once only.

Note
Reactions and/or sensitivities in this area could relate to arthritis in the foot or blood pressure disorders. Only experienced therapists should treat if an existing heart condition is present.

CARDIAC/HEART REFLEX - LEFT FOOT ONLY

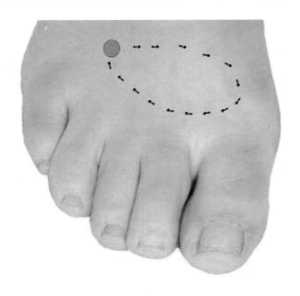

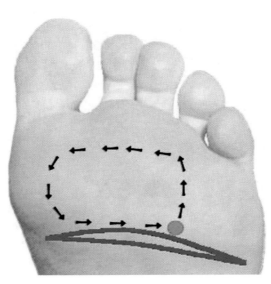

23. Liver Reflex – RIGHT FOOT ONLY

Location
Zone 3 to Zone 5
Right Foot

Area
Upper Abdomen

Digit
Thumb

Technique
Caterpillar Walk

Hold
Foot Wrap.

Treatment
Across upper abdomen, between diaphragm and waist. Place the thumb across the upper abdomen in line with toe three. Caterpillar walk across the area from Zone 3 to Zone 5. Do as many movements as necessary until the upper two thirds of the area between the diaphragm and waist is treated. Then treat entire area again but this time work the liver from Zone 5 to Zone 3.

How Often
Once in each direction. If a reactive reflex or a related condition presenting, do the treatment once more.

Note
The liver is also treated in the upper abdomen, sequence number 21.

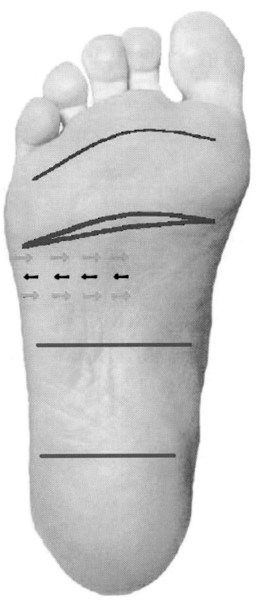

23. Spleen Reflex – LEFT FOOT ONLY

Location
Zone 4 – Zone 5

Area
Sole - left foot only
between diaphragm line and waist line

Digit
Thumb

Technique
Caterpillar Walk

Hold
Foot Wrap

Treatment
Across upper abdomen, between diaphragm and waist. Place the thumb across the upper abdomen in line with toe three. Caterpillar walk across the area from Zone 4 to Zone 5. Do as many movements as necessary until the upper two thirds of the area between the diaphragm and waist is treated. Then treat entire area again but this time work the spleen from Zone 5 to Zone 4.

How Often
Do the movement once only. If a reactive reflex or a related condition presenting, do the treatment three more times.

Note
When treating patients who are receiving chemotherapy, treat the spleen twice more (total six times).

SPLEEN REFLEX – LEFT FOOT ONLY

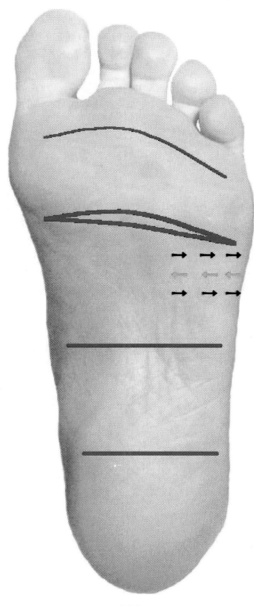

24. Stomach/Duodenum/Pancreas – RIGHT FOOT

Location
Zone 1 to Zone 2

Area
Sole between Diaphragm Line
And Waist Line

Digit
Thumb

Technique
Caterpillar Walk

Hold
Foot Wrap

Treatment
Put your thumb on the medial edge of the foot directly under the diaphragm line, pointing towards the outer edge (lateral). Caterpillar walk across the foot from Zone 1 to Zone 2. Continue working in this manner to cover upper two thirds of area between diaphragm line and waist line. Swap hands over and this time work the same area but in the opposite direction, i.e. from Zone 2 to Zone 1.

How Often
Once. If a reactive reflex or a related condition presenting, do the treatment once more.

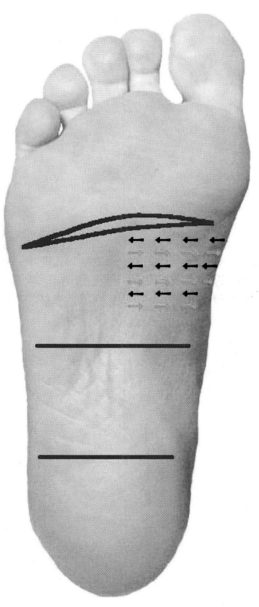

24. Stomach, Pancreas, Duodenum - LEFT FOOT

Location
Zone 1 – Zone 3

Area
Sole between diaphragm line and waist line.

Digit
Thumb

Technique
Caterpillar Walk

Hold
Foot Wrap or Sole Support

Treatment
Put the thumb on the medial edge of the foot, directly under the diaphragm line, pointing towards the outer edge (lateral). Caterpillar walk across the foot from Zone 1 to Zone 3. Continue working in this manner to cover upper two thirds of area between diaphragm line and waist line. Swap hands and this time work the same area but in the opposite direction, i.e. from Zone 3 to Zone 1.

How Often
Do movement once only. If a reactive reflex or a related condition presenting, do the treatment once more.

Note
Duodenum reflex in Zone 1 on this foot is very small.

STOMACH, PANCREAS, DUODENUM - LEFT FOOT

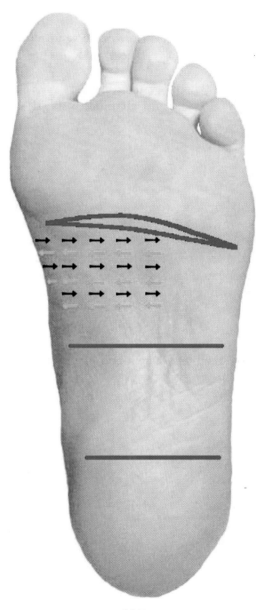

25. Lower Abdomen - Small Intestine

Location
Zone 1 to Zone 5

Area
Between Waist Line and Pelvic Floor Line

Digit
Thumb

Technique
Caterpillar Walk

Hold
Foot Wrap.

Treatment
Across lower abdomen, between waist and pelvic floor line. Place the thumb across the lower abdomen in line with toe one. Caterpillar walk across the area from Zone 1 to Zone 5. Do as many movements as necessary until the area between the waist line and pelvic floor line is treated. Then treat entire area again but this time work from Zone 5 to Zone 1.

How Often
Once in each direction. If a reactive reflex or a related condition presenting, do the treatment once more.

LOWER ABDOMEN - SMALL INTESTINE

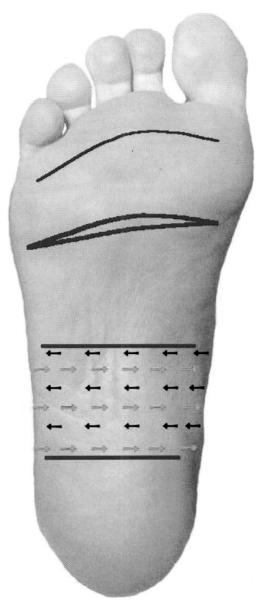

26. Lower Back, Gluteals, Pelvis, Sciatic (Support Reflex)

Location
Zone 1 to Zone 5

Area
Hard Heel Pad

Digit
Thumb

Technique
Caterpillar Walk

Hold
Heel Grip

Treatment

i)   Caterpillar walk across the heel pad from the inner edge,
       Zone 1, to the outer edge, Zone 5, starting at the pelvic floor line.
       Work downwards to the base of the heel. Do as many movements
       as necessary in order to cover the area.

ii)   Caterpillar walk up from the base of the heel to the pelvic floor.
       Work from Zone 1 to Zone 5. Do as many movements as
       necessary to cover the area.

How Often
Do movement once in each direction. If reactive reflex or a related
condition presenting, do the treatment once more in each direction.

LOWER BACK, GLUTEALS, PELVIS, SCIATIC
(SUPPORT REFLEX)

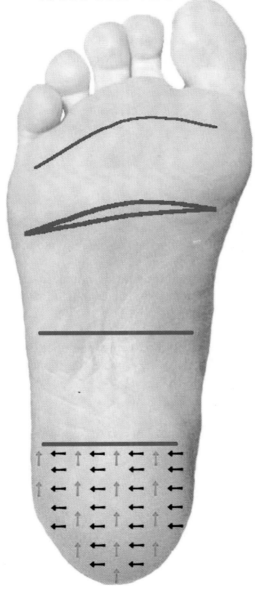

27. Sciatic Support

Location
Zone 1 to Zone 5

Area
Back of Lower Leg
Calf Muscle (*gastrocnemius*)

Digit
Whole Hand

Technique
i) Pressure Slide
ii) Squeeze and Push

Hold
Heel Grip – Foot Wrap

Treatment

i)   Put the working palm uppermost against the leg, slide towards the knee, while keeping the pressure up into the muscle.

ii)   Close the working hand around the calf muscle. Squeeze, release, move forward. Work in this manner until the calf muscle is treated.

How Often
Do movement number (i) and movement number (ii) twice each. If a reactive reflex or a related condition presenting, do the movement twice more.

Note
If client has a varicose vein do not squeeze but gently stroke up the back of the leg.

SCIATIC SUPPORT

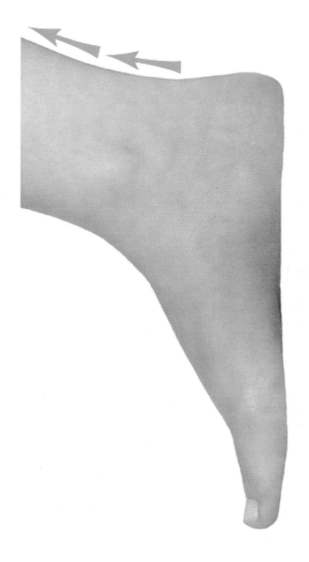

28. Sciatic Reflex

Location
Zone 5 to Zone 1

Area
Behind both ankles and across centre of heel pad

Digit
Thumb

Technique
Caterpillar Walk

Hold
Foot Wrap or Heel Grip

Treatment
Work down behind outer ankle, across centre of hard heel pad, up behind inner ankle bone.
Rest the fingers of the working hand across the leg (in the area of the ankles). Put the thumb of this hand behind the outer ankle bone, the tip pointing towards the heel.
Use the thumb to caterpillar walk down the foot to the heel, turn the thumb and work across the centre of the hard heel pad, from Zone 5 to Zone 1. Turn thumb again, this time work up behind the inner ankle bone to the top of the ankle. Change hands and repeat movement in opposite direction.

How Often
Do the movement once in each direction, if reactive reflex or a related condition presenting, do the treatment twice more in each direction.

Note
In order to treat the inner ankle area it may be necessary to change the working and holding hands around.

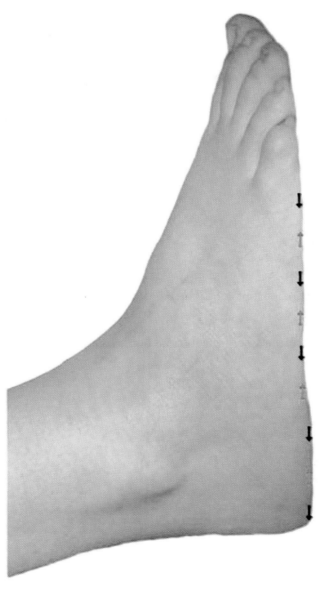

31. Additional Treatment for Problem Joint Areas

<u>A: Elbow</u>

Location	*Area*
Zone 5 to	Bite down from the
Zone 4-5	metatarsophalangeal joint on the
	lateral edge.

Digit	*Technique*
Thumb	Caterpillar Walks - in small bites
	Pressure Circles (Rotations)

Hold
Heel Grip

Treatment
Caterpillar walk for 3 small bites down the outside (lateral) edge of the foot, from the base of the little toe. Then caterpillar walk for 3 small bites up on to the top of the foot. Give 3 deep pressure circles/rotations.

How Often
Do the movement once in acute conditions. Twice for chronic conditions.

Note
Left hand work on right foot.
Right hand work on left foot.

31. Additional Treatment for Problem Joint Areas

B: Knee

Location
Zone 5 to
Zone 4-5

Area
Lateral protrusion (base of 5th
metatarsal)

Digit
Thumb

Technique
Caterpillar Walks - in small bites
Pressure Circles (Rotations)

Hold
Heel Grip

Treatment
Caterpillar walk down the lateral edge of the foot, from the base of the
little toe, until you reach the protrusion mid-way down the edge of the
foot (base of 5th metatarsal). Then caterpillar walk for 5 small bites up
onto the top of the foot (in line with gap between toe 4 and toe 5). Give
5 deep pressure circles (rotations). Next turn thumb and caterpillar
walk towards the toes. Just before reaching the elbow reflex stop and
give a further 5 pressure circles.

How Often
Do movement once in acute conditions. Twice in chronic conditions.

31. Additional Treatment for Problem Joint Areas

C: Hip

Location
Zone 5

Area
From just below the protrusion
(heel side) to tip of heel

Digit
4 Fingers

Technique
All finger Caterpillar Walk

Hold
Ankle/Achilles Support

Treatment
While supporting the foot with one hand, cup the heel in the other hand
and use all fingers of this hand to caterpillar walk up the outside of the
foot.

How Often
Once for acute conditions. Twice for chronic conditions.

ADDITIONAL TREATMENT FOR
PROBLEM JOINT AREAS

A. Elbow

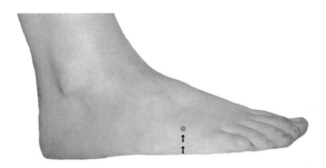

B. Knee

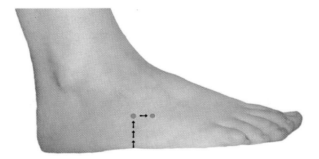

C. Hip

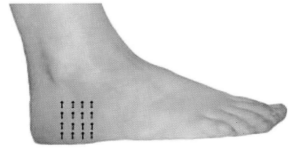

32. Rectum/Anus/Pelvis

Location
Zone 1 – Zone 5

Area
Around outside edge of heel

Digit
Thumb

Technique
Caterpillar Walk

Hold
Foot Wrap or Heel Grip

Treatment
Using the pelvic floor line as a guide to start and finish movement, work in a horseshoe shape around the outer edge of the heel. Put thumb on lateral edge of foot, level with pelvic floor line, pointing down towards heel, caterpillar walk around the heel to the corresponding point on the medial side (inside). Here give three distinct pressure circles on the rectum/anus support reflex.

How Often
Do each movement twice. If a reactive reflex or a related condition presenting, do the treatment once more.

Note
If haemorrhoids present be gentle with pressure circles/rotations.

RECTUM/ANUS/PELVIS

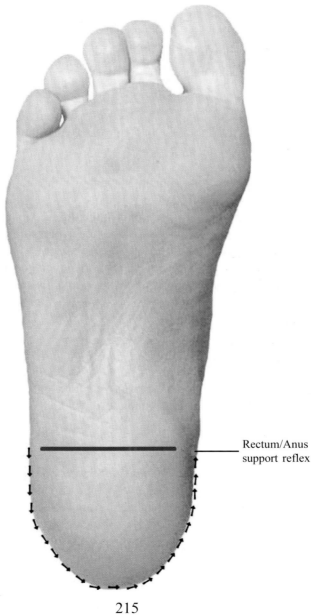

Rectum/Anus
support reflex

33. Kidney, Ureter Tubes

Location
Between Zone 2
& Zone 3

Area
Sole of foot

Digit
Thumb

Technique
Deep pressure circles or
foot rotated onto thumb

Hold
Foot Wrap

Treatment
i)   Put the distal joint (first joint) of the thumb, tip towards toes,
       straddling the waist line. Give two deep pressure circles. Release
       thumb for a second, then repeat movement.
ii)   Swivel thumb, tip towards heel, work down the foot on the ureter
       tube reflex to the pelvic floor line, then continue the movement
       up onto the soft mound on the inside (medial side) of the foot
       (bladder).

How Often
Do each movement once. If a reactive reflex or a related condition
presenting, do the treatment twice more.

Note
Use left hand on right kidney and right hand on left kidney. Be aware
that some therapists work down the foot on the ureter tubes at an
acute angle, crossing to the bladder before reaching the pelvic floor.
Having researched both methods, I find working to the pelvic floor
area before swivelling the thumb towards bladder to be the more
effective method.

KIDNEY, URETER TUBES

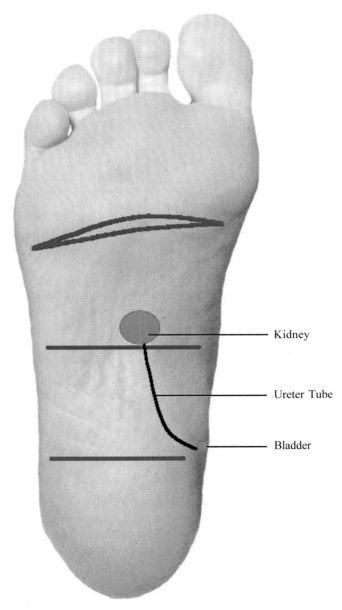

Kidney

Ureter Tube

Bladder

217

34. Bladder

Location
Zone 1

Area
Inner side of foot in a soft mound
big toe side of pelvic floor line

Digit
Thumb

Technique
i)   Three pressure circles
ii)   Three or four (depending on foot
      size) Caterpillar Walks, radiating
      outwards from bladder in
      general direction of big toe

Hold
Foot Wrap

Treatment
i)   Place the thumb in the centre of the soft flesh area and give
      three deep pressure circles
ii)   Keep the thumb in position, then make three or four short
      caterpillar walks outwards from the bladder in the general
      direction of the big toe. Slide back to the centre in between
      each walk.

How Often
Do the movement once. If a reactive reflex or a related condition
presenting, do the treatment twice more.

Note
You may swap hands to do the caterpillar walks.
If the bladder reflex (mound) is not very clear on the inside of the foot,
press your thumb into the sole close to the pelvic floor line. This action
tends to make the bladder reflex more visible as a mound on the side of
the foot.

BLADDER

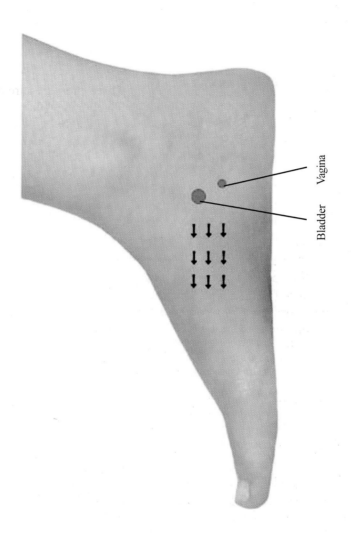

35. Adrenals

Location
Between Zone 1 and
Zone 2

Area
Sole in line with toe 2

Digit
Thumb

Technique
Hook in and back up
Bee sting-like action

Hold
Foot Wrap or Sole Support

Treatment
Put one thumb on kidney reflex (to act as location guide). Bring second
thumb, pointing in the opposite direction (towards the heel). The nails
of both thumbs should be almost parallel.

i)   Remove the thumb from the kidney location point
ii)   Press the adrenal reflex thumb deeply into the sole
iii)   Keeping the thumb in contact, bend the first joint, so the knuckle
        is visible; drop your wrist at the same time. This will cause an
        action similar to a bee delivering a sting (hook in, back up). Flatten
        and hook three distinct times.

How Often
Do the movement once, If a reactive reflex or a related condition
presenting, do the treatment twice more. If very sensitive or a severe
related problem exists, return at the end of the full treatment and treat
the reflex once more.

ADRENALS

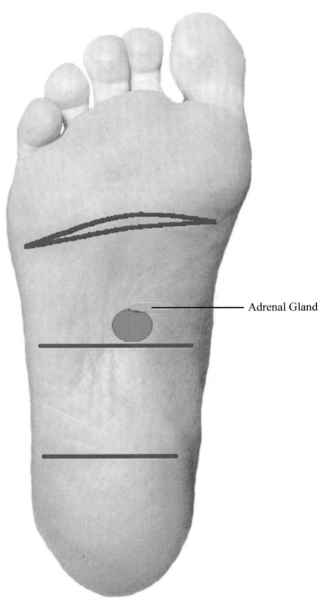

Adrenal Gland

36. Uterus Female, Prostate Male

Location
Zone 1

Area
Medial side of foot, midway between the high point in the centre of the ankle bone and the back tip of the heel.

Digit
Thumb
or Index Finger

Technique
Pressure Circle/Rotation
Stroke

Hold
Foot Wrap – lean foot outwards

Treatment
Draw an imaginary line from the high point in the centre of the inner ankle bone to the back corner (tip) of the heel.
Place your thumb/index finger in the centre of the line and work around the area, making a number of distinct circular/rotating movements. Work in a pattern to cover an area about the size of a man's thumb nail.

How Often
Do the movement on the area once. If reactive reflex or a related condition presenting, including infertility, do the movement twice more.

Note
If IUD fitted or pregnant, stroke the uterus area rather than press.

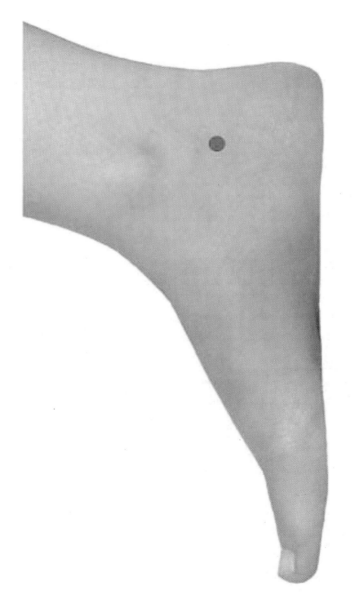

37. Ovary Female, Testicle Male

Location
Zone 5

Area
Lateral side of foot, midway between the high point in the centre of the ankle bone and the back tip of the heel.

Digit
Thumb
or Index Finger

Technique
Pressure Circle/Rotation

Hold
Foot Wrap – lean foot inwards

Treatment
Draw an imaginary line from the high point in the centre of the outer ankle bone to the back corner (tip) of the heel.
Place your thumb/index finger in the centre of the line and work around the area, making a number of distinct circular/rotating movements. Work in a pattern to cover an area about the size of a man's thumb nail.

How Often
Do the movement on the area once. If related problems exist, including infertility, do the movement twice more.

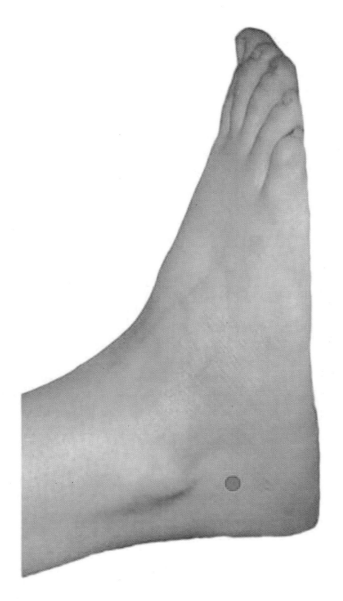

38. Fallopian/Uterine Tubes, Female; Vas Deferens, Male

Location
Zone 5 to Zone 1

Area
Imaginary line from outer to inner ankle, stretching across the foot in line with the lowest point of each ankle bone.

Digit
Thumb or
Index Finger

Technique
Caterpillar Walk

Hold
Foot Wrap

Treatment
Use the thumb or index finger (whichever is most comfortable for you) to caterpillar walk across the foot from the ovary reflex under the outer ankle to the uterus reflex under the inner ankle.

How Often
Do the movement three times. If reactive reflex or related condition presenting, such as the existence of fertility problems, do the movement a further three times. Work firstly ovary to uterus three times and then three times uterus to ovary. Finally work three times from ovary to uterus.

FALLOPIAN/UTERINE TUBES, FEMALE;
VAS DEFERENS, MALE

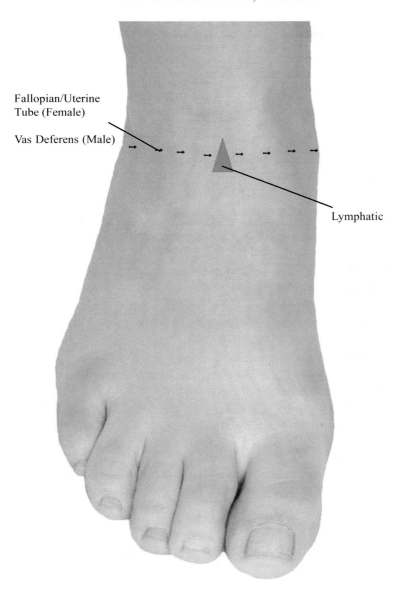

Fallopian/Uterine
Tube (Female)

Vas Deferens (Male)

Lymphatic

39. Hip – Lymphatics – Inguinals - Pelvic (Groin) Area

Location
Zone 1 and Zone 5

Area
Behind, under, in front of outer and inner ankle bone (horseshoe shape)

Digit
Thumb

Technique
Caterpillar Walk
Slide Movement

Hold
Foot Wrap:
Grip on medial aspect (inside) when treating the outer ankle. Grip on lateral (outside) when treating inner ankle.

Treatment
i)   Put your thumb on the outer edge of the heel, it should be pointing upwards towards the leg.
ii)   Caterpillar walk up behind the ankle to the top of the bone. Hold the pressure for a count of five.
iii)   Keeping the thumb in contact, slide back to the bottom of the ankle bone. The professional may prefer to turn the thumb and caterpillar walk instead of slide.
iv)   Caterpillar walk around the bone, then up in front of the ankle. At the top of the ankle bone, hold the pressure for a count of five. Slide back to bottom of ankle.
v)   Caterpillar walk across foot/leg crease line – repeat movement on inner ankle.

How Often
Do movement twice each side. If a reactive reflex or a related condition presenting, do the treatment twice more on each side.

Note
Reactive reflexes behind the ankle may relate to chronic constipation, sciatic or hip problems. Underneath the ankle may also relate to a hip problem.

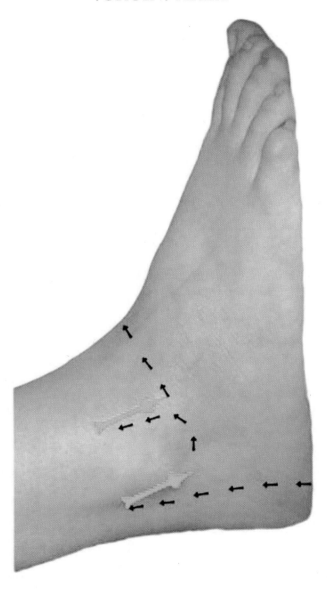

40. Breast - Lymphatics - Sternum

Location
Zone 1 to Zone 4

Area
Dorsum of foot
From base of toes to diaphragm

Digit
Index Finger

Technique
i)   Caterpillar walk movement,
     Each step followed by a gentle
     hook in and back up technique.
ii) Gentle hook in technique,
     followed by a backward walk.

Hold
Sole Support

Treatment
i)   Put the index finger on the top of the foot at the base of big toe.
     Make a small caterpillar walk forward, then hook in and pull
     back. Work in this manner down the foot to the diaphragm line.
ii) Next work back along the same line to the base of big toe. The
     movement this time will be to hook in and pull back, then to
     flatten finger and slide back one step then hook in again. Continue
     to work in this manner, doing as many movements as necessary
     to treat the area between Zone 1 and Zone 4.

How Often
Do the movement once. If a reactive reflex or a related condition
presenting, do the treatment once more.

Note
Reflexes of the lungs, lymphatics, ribs, sternum and breast may be
reactive within this area. Half zone 1 relates to the sternum. Between
zones 2 and 3 relates to lymphatics of thoracic. Zone 2 to 4 relates to
breast. Work this area with a more superficial movement on the way
back to the toes.

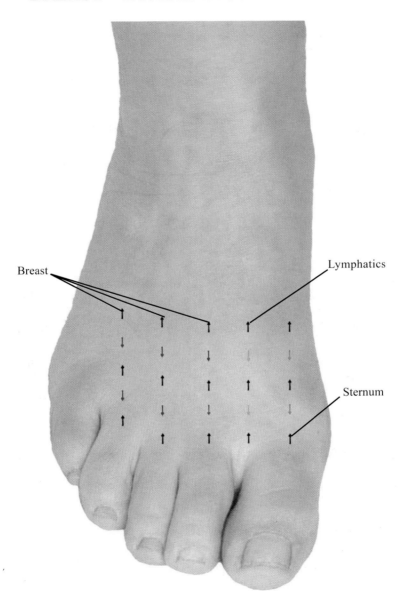

Breast

Lymphatics

Sternum

41. General Body Boost – BOTH FEET

TREAT LEFT FOOT FIRST AND RIGHT FOOT SECOND

Location
Zone 1 – Zone 5
Start on left foot

Area
Sides and top of foot
between toes and ankle

Digit
All fingers of both hands

Technique
Finger Caterpillar Walk

Hold
Thumbs rest on sole
Fingers working on top

Treatment
i)   Use both hands for this movement.
ii)   Put your right hand on the outside edge of the foot and your left
       hand on the inside edge. The fingers of each hand should be
       pointing towards the top of the foot. The thumbs should be resting
       on the sole.
iii)   Caterpillar walk all fingers towards each other until they lock
       together on the top of the foot.
iv)   Slide back to the edge of the foot and move the hands up a little
       towards the toes.
v)   Continue to work in this manner until the area between the toes
       and the ankle is treated.
vi)   Move to the right foot and treat it in a similar manner.

How Often
Do the movement once on each foot. However, if used for general
relaxation, it can be done up to 4 more times on each foot.

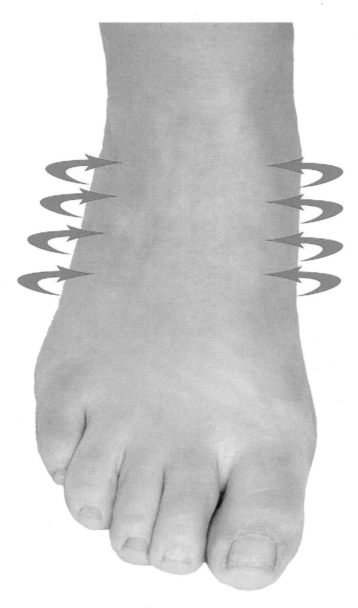

42. Colon - Ileocaecal Valve - Appendix

Location	*Area*
Between Zone 4 - Zone 5	From pelvic line to mid-way
Both feet	between waist and diaphragm
Zone 1 - Zone 5	- Across right foot from between Z4
Both Feet	& Z5 to Z1.
	- Across left foot from Z1 to between
	Z4 & Z5
	- Down left foot from between Z4
	& Z5 to pelvic line
	- Across left foot to Zone 1
	- Down left foot to tip of heel Z1

Digit	*Technique*
Thumb	Caterpillar Walk
	Pressure Circles/Rotations

Hold

Foot Wrap. (Remember to swap hands around on the LEFT FOOT, descending colon).

Treatment

i) Put thumb on sole just above pelvic line, between Zone 4 and Zone 5, with tip pointing towards Zone 1. Give four distinct pressure circles/rotations on appendix and ileocaecal valve.

ii) Turn thumb to point towards toes. Caterpillar walk up foot to midway between waist line and diaphragm line. Turn thumb (hepatic flexor) and work to Zone 1 across transverse colon.

iii) Change to left foot. Continue to work across this foot (transverse colon) to between Zone 4 and Zone 5. Turn thumb (splenic flexure) and work down (descending colon) to pelvic line.

iv) Turn thumb again and work towards Zone 1. However you will stop in line with Zone 3 and 4. Turn tip of thumb towards the heel and give 3 distinct deep pressure circles/rotations on the sigmoid colon. Return thumb to previous position and continue to work towards Zone 1.

v)   At the edge of the foot, just underneath the bladder, give 3 pressure circles (rotations) on the rectum/anus helper reflex, then caterpillar walk down the rectum to the tip of the heel and give 3 pressure circles (rotations) on the anus reflex.

How Often

Do the movement three times. If a reactive reflex or a related condition presenting, do the treatment twice more.

Note

When colon/digestive inflammatory problems exist, commence with a light pressure increasing to the client's tolerance level.

COLON - ILEOCAECAL VALVE - APPENDIX

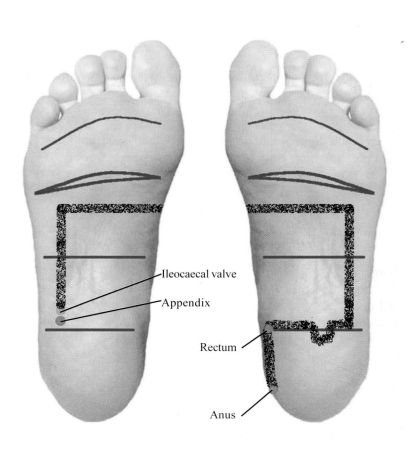

Ileocaecal valve

Appendix

Rectum

Anus

CONCLUDE THE TREATMENT

Return to treat reflexes as necessary

- **TREAT DIAPHRAGM**

- **TREAT SOLAR PLEXUS**

- **GIVE RELAXATION MASSAGE**

- **GIVE A GLASS OF WATER**

- **GIVE AFTERCARE**
  (i.e. self help; see GP; drink at least 3 glasses of water daily).

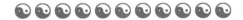

Some slight changes have been made to the method of treatment described in this 5th edition compared with previously published works. All changes follow detailed comparisons and analysis of treatment outcomes on a minimum of 500 clients over the past five years.

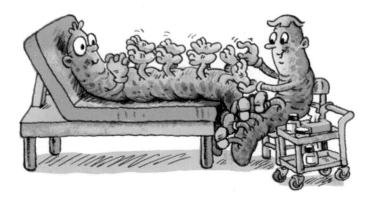

SOME COMMON QUESTIONS ANSWERED

1.   **What is Reflexology?**

The science that deals with the principle that there are reflex points on the hands and feet which correspond to all parts of the body's glands, organs and structures.

2.   **What are the benefits?**

We have four main areas to look at:

1.   To increase blood and lymph flow
2.   To relieve stress and tension
3.   To promote nerve energy
4.   To help the body maintain a state of balance

3.   **What does a cheese smell to the feet indicate?**

The body is congested with waste and toxins (often constipated).

4.   **What does an Acetone smell indicate to the therapist?**

This smell will suggest a possible urinary disorder, not necessarily serious. It is sometimes evident in the diabetic.

5.   **How much pressure do I use?**

1.   Depends on the type of foot being treated
2.   Depends on the sensitivity of the client being treated
3.   A heavy foot would need deep pressure
4.   A slim, delicate foot would need a light pressure
5.   A sick or frail person would need a light pressure
6.   A child would need light pressure
7.   A good guide is to observe the client's face
8.   Ask for feedback

6. **How many treatments?**

In this stressed world of ours, ideally the therapist would like to recommend six to eight treatments. However, I believe one treatment not only to be beneficial but financially realistic, especially when not dealing with a specific problem. The number of treatments and duration of each will depend on a number of factors, health and wealth being key considerations in recommendations.

7. **Do the chronic condition and the acute condition react to the same number of treatments?**

No. The chronic condition will usually need more treatments before there are noticeable signs of improvement. The acute condition may require less treatments while the chronic condition may require many, but each person is individual and reactions and outcomes will vary.

8. **How many treatments should I give in order to establish the effectiveness of Reflexology?**

This is a difficult question to answer. However as a general guide, it is best not to continue treatment after the third or fourth treatment if the client is unable to report any changes.

9. **How often do I treat?**

This very much depends on the client's condition and financial situation but once a week is ideal for most people as the reactions to treatment do not always show immediately, but can take up to three or four days in some cases. As a general guide the more sick the patient/client, the more realistic is a weekly treatment. Should the reactions be very strong then the recipient of the treatment can be made to feel worse, giving them a greater burden to carry.

10. **Are there any circumstances when I would treat more often than once per week?**

Yes. There are conditions that would benefit from a treatment more often than once a week but do assess your client very carefully.

A very fit client who suffers a sprain/strain could benefit from two or even more treatments in the space of one week.

An otherwise fit/healthy client who is suffering from P.M.S. and/or pain can benefit from a twice weekly treatment but proceed with caution as P.M.S. may show signs of getting worse before it gets better (strong healing reaction). The client would always be advised of this possible reaction (these clients have always been amongst my most successful).

11.   **Does Reflexology hurt?**

No. Reflexology should not hurt but some areas on the foot may feel tender or different, even a little uncomfortable (therapist adjust pressure).

12.   **What does it mean if the client complains to the therapist of a bruising dull pain on the area being treated?**

This reaction seems to be experienced by those with more chronic conditions. However the therapist should establish that there is no injury to the foot in that area.

13.   **What does it mean if the client complains of a very sharp pain, a sticking pain or a cutting pain in the area being treated?**

This type of reaction tends to be felt by those suffering with an acute condition but as always, the therapist would ensure that there was no injury to the foot.

14.   **What do I do if the client reaction is:**

   i)   *Hands perspiring*
           Continue the treatment but reduce your pressure
           Cause: nervousness, healing through obvious elimination.

   ii)   *All over perspiration*
           Stop the treatment. Hold the foot/hand for a little while then continue to treat but reduce the depth of pressure. Do plenty of relaxation strokes.
           Cause: A very strong reaction to treatment. Healing through obvious elimination.

   iii)   *An abnormal feeling of coldness, especially in the limbs, perhaps accompanied by listlessness.*
           Stop and cover client with an extra blanket or towel making sure that he/she is warm. Stroke the foot/hand gently for a few minutes. Return to Reflexology but this time make sure that the pressure is very

gentle. Instead of the normal routine, clear all zones, treat the solar plexus, the kidney ureters and bladder, then treat the adrenal and the colon. Follow this with treatment of the solar plexus and a full foot/hand massage.

Cause: A very strong reaction to treatment.

15. What are your views on treating cancer patients?

Reflexology can be part of the core package a patient suffering with cancer receives and can be integrated into their orthodox treatment. It is recommended that the patient's treatment centre is aware they are receiving reflexology, indeed many hospitals and hospices now offer reflexology to their patients.

Terminally ill patients will benefit from an urgent care treatment. Some will enjoy further treatment on painful or problem areas and a final foot or hand massage.

Cancer patients who are feeling a little fragile will benefit from this routine for the first treatment session. Thereafter a normal treatment will encourage healing and well being. Pressure used should be lighter than normal (be aware of tendency to bruise).

Chemotherapy patients will benefit from a full reflexology treatment one or two days prior to their treatment and a zone walk as soon as possible after the chemotherapy (same day preferably).

Note

All professionals considering working with cancer patients should undertake specific training.

16. Would you treat a person with a fever?

No. Not as a rule. A fever might suggest a contagious condition. It may also put an extra burden on the healing process with which the body could not cope. However in recurrent fever with no apparent medical cause (especially in children) to treat the pituitary gland x 4 in the first hour followed by a general endocrine treatment has been known to produce good results. Allow two hours to elapse before returning to treatment.

17. What can you tell me about a corn on the foot?

Corns are patches of hard skin which become dense in the centre. They can cause intense pain, due to pressure. Corns are found most frequently on toes 1, 3 and 4 and appear as a result of pressure from footwear. This protective shield will indicate to the therapist a possible reflex disturbance in the zone/reflex.

18.   What can you tell me about a build up of hard skin?

The foot forms hard skin to protect it from rough surfaces. This can be a ridge on the sole of a shoe, walking around bare foot or the natural posture and stance of a particular person. Hard skin that is flexible poses little threat to reflex disturbances but the thick, horny, inflexible skin often found on the heel, ball of the foot and the edge of the big toe, can indicate energy blockages.

19.   Can you remind me about the necessity of the consultation card?

- To establish there are no contra indications to the treatment.

- To assess the client's physical and mental state.

- To show a genuine interest and establish their expectations.

- To ensure that our therapy is holistic and meets clients' needs.

- To ensure that we give the best possible treatment for each client.

- To establish that Reflexology is the most suitable treatment.

- To refer client to a therapist with the appropriate skills or to a medically qualified practitioner.

20.   What physiological changes are likely to occur when the client talks during the treatment

Talking takes energy. Conversation about people puts the visual imagination to work, altering brain wave rhythms in the process. Thoughts are coloured by emotions and this in turn influences brain waves, dividing the brain's reflex action. Conversation may interfere with blood circulation since thoughts and emotions cause vascular change, dilating or contracting blood vessels and altering normal rhythms of contraction and expansion. If conversation is related to the present, the client/patient can focus on the sensations being felt at that moment. However the therapist must never loose sight of the fact that one of his/her greatest assets will be listening skills. Clients will sometimes like to talk about their lives and problems. The therapist must not be judgemental though it is possible to perhaps suggest a different approach to the problem. The client's new approach to life may then help the body to function in a state of balance.

21. **How should I respond when the client asks, 'What exactly are you treating'?**

The Reflexologist treats the whole person through stimulating the nerve endings, the energy channels and vascular flow to the various organs and structures of the body which are reflected in miniature on the feet and hands.

22. **Reflexology balances and revitalises. What do you mean?**

Illness, stress, tension and fatigue can each have the effect of causing body disharmony (imbalance). Energy is wasted fighting the problem or struggling mentally with negative attitudes. Reflexology encourages the body's own energy flow and as the body and mind regain their balance they can work more efficiently.

23. **What if the bladder reflex is not just a puffy area on the side of the foot but stretches almost onto the sole.**

There are a number of reasons, one of which is that this could be normal for this person. It could in some cases indicate a full bladder, dehydration, or even a prolapsed bladder. A professional therapist would not make the latter statement to a client/patient.

24. **An alcoholic asked me for help. Is there any point in treating?**

Yes indeed! Do say that you will help but that there will be a joint involvement in the result. Do not treat the client whilst he/she is in a state of alcohol abuse/drunk. It is possible to encourage the client to gradually reduce their intake. In all cases I have treated I have found severe reactions on the entire endocrine system and I have given more treatment to the sensitive areas, but always in conjunction with a complete treatment. Over the course of the years I have successfully treated three alcoholics who, once the course of Reflexology had started, had no other form of treatment (various therapies had been tried previously). Professional therapists should have support and further training to work in this field.

25. **The client is feeling unwell but no sensitivity is found during treatment. Why?**

Possible causes for lack of reactions:

■ The pressure is too light for the size/bulk of foot

- Medication has in some way anaesthetised the reflexes

- The client has a high pain threshold

- There is a lot of congestion in the feet that needs clearing first

- The client's perception of pain

26. When you say press, how long does the therapist press for?

The therapist should count "one, two, three" distinctly (but not out loud) during the hold for each press. Each press should last between 2 and 3 seconds.

27. What are the likely results of working for too long in any one session?

To work too long or indeed too deeply leads to the possibility of over stimulation which can cause excessive elimination and discomfort. This in turn, can make the client feel that the Reflexology is too unpleasant for them.

28. What are the likely results of a treatment that is too short?

In this case the body is not provided with sufficient stimulus to mobilise its own healing powers.

29. What is the energy? Where does it come from?

A Chinese belief is that the whole functioning of the body and mind depends on the normal flow of energies which they call life force or chi, pronounced 'Chee', (in modern translation/interpretation sometimes called Qi – pronounced 'Ki'). Chi is a universal energy which pervades everything. We can neither see nor feel it, in much the same way as we cannot see or feel radio waves or ultra violet.
The energy in the body comes from the air we breathe and the food we eat. (There is no doubt that when we eat nutritionally rich food we are also taking in energy). Strong energy protects the body, acting as a defence system. The language of western medicine refers to this as a high resistance. If the chi is weak then the resistance is lowered which can result in illness of body or mind. Whether we think in terms of immune response or of chi, once illness has set in our inner resistance is of great importance in determining how well we cope and recover. Reflexologists, through using their various methodologies, are each aiming to strengthen and balance the energy flow. Reflex points might be considered here as energy junctions that respond to pressure.

30.   Why do books and charts differ in relation to reflex and zonal areas?

The body's organs and structures are always more or less in the same place but obviously muscle tone, age changes and heredity influences do have a bearing. All reflexologists agree with this statement. They further agree that no part of the body has its own precise compartment; all parts are forced to dwell in shared accommodation with their neighbours, muscles, blood vessels, nerves and even other organs. A simple analogy could be packing a drawer in your bedroom or your suitcase to go on holiday, there is space for everything and everything has a space. However in Reflexology the therapist is packing the contents of the entire wardrobe into the bedroom drawer or holiday suitcase. In other words, when the therapist is reflecting the entire body onto the feet, each point of reflexion has to be very small, in some cases even minute. Therefore experience has taught that to support some of the reflex points with helper areas that are either system or zonal linked will improve the overall value of the Reflexology treatment.

The reason why there tends to be some slight differences in reflex or zonal points is simple. It depends on whether the author includes all or most reflex points and helper areas or works only with some of the points that they consider important in order to gain the desired effect. For example some writers point out the inner ear only, whereas I put in all the ear treatment points and helper areas. What the student/therapist needs to be sure of is that the anatomical mapping and/or the zonal mapping is being adhered to by the writer and that the originator of the text or chart has the knowledge and experience to produce material. One example of anatomical mis-mapping in reflexology is, for example, the stomach being placed in the chest area above the diaphragm line. Another and more obvious one is when the breasts/mammary glands are placed on the chart below the waist line. It should be noted that a number of text books will use a combination of reflex and zonal points to gain the best response. Therapists who have worked for many years will always write books or publish charts based on their own clinical findings and documented notes, but there will to me always be a relationship in the writings. There are writers who have remained faithful to the original ideas and have not done independent studies or progressed forward.
There are one or two books available that do differ quite considerably from the accepted norm. These books are, in my opinion, totally unsuitable for the student and for the professional therapist, in that they bear little or no relationship to anatomical mapping or zonal relationships. Only the writings of the experienced therapist will be of value to the student of Reflexology. The qualified therapist will have the knowledge to be selective.

31.   Should I treat during Pregnancy?

During pregnancy we are dealing with two lives, not just one and unless the therapist has specialised training relative to pregnancy, no treatment should be given but a referral should be made to a maternity reflexologist.

245

Reflexology is known, amongst other things, to relieve morning sickness and back aches as well as boosting energy levels. Self-help should be advised by a maternity reflexologist.

32. Should the therapist give home care advice relevant to pregnancy?

Home care at this time can be very beneficial. However, I would recommend that the advice be given only by a suitably qualified therapist who can assess the client's understanding of that advice prior to the mother doing self treatment.

33. Is reflexology beneficial during labour?

Reflexology during labour has many recorded benefits and is becoming increasingly popular in many countries throughout the world. Experience has demonstrated a more relaxed mother, shorter labour, less need for pain relief and increased energy. Some research has also demonstrated the benefits of treatment in cases of retained placenta. Treatment and self help advice should be given by a professional.

34. Is Reflexology an appropriate treatment for infertility? Can it help?

The reason for infertility will obviously have a bearing on the benefits or otherwise of reflexology. In order for reflexology to be successful there would need to be a possibility for success. Ideally treatment would be given on a weekly basis, if this is not possible then treatment a few days prior to ovulation and/or during the week of ovulation would be best. A full treatment given to both partners by a professional therapist would increase the chances of conception. The professional therapist could also offer advice on self help treatment.

There is much evidence to prove the worth of reflexology beyond coincidence in this area. A full treatment is essential with emphasis on endocrine and reproductive glands and the spine (spleen, liver,stomach to encourage nutrient-rich circulation)

35. Can reflexology be given during I.V.F?

Yes, by an experienced therapist who is aiming to balance the systems and improve circulation. Too much pressure and prolonged treatment will over stimulate.

36.   Can you give us a little more information about treating children?

It is important to note that it is a legal requirement as well as an ethical obligation to seek medical assistance for any undiagnosed conditions in children. Do not attempt to treat anything that may need medical attention.

Children can respond very well to Reflexology treatment. The therapist should bear in mind that the child can have similar reactions to the therapy as would an adult, so treatment pressure, pace and duration would be judged accordingly.

The small child with little or no verbal communication skills will sometimes respond to sensitive reflexes by pulling the foot away and/or fidgeting, or even by clinging tightly to the parent or guardian.

The slightly older child (four-six years of age) is often chatty and usually happy to be told exactly what is happening; they are, in most cases very accurate in their verbal response to a sensitive reflex.

The child of eight or nine years upwards requires that the therapist be particularly observant in noting changes in expression. At this age conditioning has often already taken place in relation to standards of acceptability with regard to complaining about levels of discomfort/hurt (the child might feel he/she ought not to). Always ask for feedback, pleasant or otherwise.

The younger teenager will often be more relaxed in the absence of a parent or guardian. While I am not suggesting that the latter be precluded from the treatment area, I have found that experience and intuition play a part in the therapist's decision to ask the parent/guardian for a little time alone with the child. This may of course be difficult, or pose its own problems, for example with opposite sexes or a first time visitor. I have found that some young people will not discuss problems in the presence of an accompanying adult, even problems such as school or peer bullying (at times the root cause of the problem).

The majority of children/teenagers are model patients/clients and love the attention of the one to one. In most cases they will confide in the therapist (don't worry; it may not happen on the first visit). The therapist should never dismiss anyone's fears let alone those of the child. All fears are real and never trivial to the one expressing them. Verbal reassurance coupled with a treatment can often work wonders.

In the above section I have chosen to mention those children who suffer no obvious handicaps but I do feel that a special mention is due to all those parents and the children who suffer a disability of any form. I have experienced the privilege of working with some such children and in all cases have been rewarded with a positive response (no matter how small). My successes have been as varied as with almost any other group: from bowel regularity and improving sleep patterns to relaxation.

37. Should children receive a full treatment routine on the first visit?

While the aim of the professional therapist will be to work towards giving a full treatment based on the child's needs, the pressure should always be lighter than that for an adult. In the baby and very young, the pressure is a little more than a stroke. However, care should be taken to ensure the movement is not ticklish or irritating, not just to the child but to any age group.

The initial treatment to assess outcomes could be the routine that is now known world wide as *'The Renée Tanner Urgent Care Routine'*. In subsequent treatments this can be built on, to accommodate the specific needs of the child, or in some cases it may be all that is needed or tolerated by the child, but especially small babies and very sick children. When treating children below the age of puberty, care should be taken not to over-stimulate the endocrine glands.

NOTE: The *Urgent Care Routine* is also suitable for adults.

38. What is the minimum age for treating babies?

There is no minimum age. Everyone, including baby benefits from human touch. Naturally in day old babies, stroking is appropriate. New babies relax, sleep better and even seem to enjoy their food following a foot stroking reflexology treatment.

A special child case study

Robert, who throughout his eight years of life in total silence had not given even one recorded smile. Not only was Robert deaf, he had the mental age of a four year old and the obvious physical disability of having only one arm. I was asked by a friend to give Robert's mother a treatment as a birthday treat. She told me about Robert and asked if I could meet with him though I did not normally make house calls I decided to make an exception and went off to meet Robert at 3:30 the next day.

I sat in the room close to the little boy for about half an hour before attempting to touch him. For most of the time he sat motionless, dwarfed by the huge armchair into which he had run and jumped upon my arrival. Though I knew Robert could not hear me, I did make attempts to communicate with him using my eyes and lips and the various toys that lay around the room.

Eventually I held his feet and stroked one leg whilst observing the expressionless eyes. Robert's mother removed one of his shoes and I removed the other. I gave a few gentle effleurage movements to both feet followed by zonal clearing. I then treated: Solar plexus, head and brain, spine, eyes, ears, Eustachian tubes and completed the treatment with more effleurage of the feet. The treatment lasted in total about ten minutes. A week later I visited the family again. Robert took up his position in the armchair and I repeated the exact process of the previous week. The only difference was that on this occasion I also massaged his hand. He squeezed my hand on two occasions when I had stopped the effleurage. This encouraged me to repeat both the foot and hand massage as it was my impression that he was enjoying the treatment.

The process was repeated in week three. This time Robert began squeezing my hand very tightly. When I had completed the treatment I playfully shook his hand with my left hand and still with a playful fashion rubbed the top of his head with my right hand. Robert moved in an effort to free himself from both my hands. While this was happening I was jerked into reality as his mother yelled out from behind me, 'He is smiling, he is smiling!' Well, Robert was not the only one in the room smiling after we realised what he was doing. Although Robert tended to ration his smiles from then on, he would actually always give a big smile in response to having his hand effleuraged. He also learned to undo and remove his shoes and socks and make it very obvious that he wanted his feet treated. The respondent was usually treated to a beautiful smile. There are many children who may benefit from your care and efforts. I cannot tell you the joy of a response even if all are not as dramatic as Robert's.

The professional can pass on expert advice to parents/ guardians on how and when to perform movements that would be beneficial to a child (or adult), either between visits to the therapist or as an alternative to professional treatments.

39.   Are all Aromatherapists qualified Reflexologists?

No. Some Aromatherapists will have undertaken a separate course to qualify them in the field of Reflexology.

40. I have been told that Reflexology is part of Aromatherapy. Is this true?

No! Some Aromatherapists do press on some Reflexology points in order to help them choose an oil for their aromatherapy treatment; but this cannot be classified as Reflexology. However fortunately this is becoming a practice less often performed by the well qualified Aromatherapist.

41. Are all Beauty Therapists Reflexologists?

No. Beauty Therapists who hold qualifications to undertake face and body treatments will have studied anatomy, physiology and massage. However this does not qualify them as Reflexologists.

42. Does the Reflexologist have to be insured?

All professional therapists should be insured.

43. How can a Therapist get insurance to practice?

Therapists gaining their training through a recognised establishment will be given details of professional bodies/societies for membership and insurance.

44. Where can I get information about courses?

By contacting one of the Reflexology organisations listed at the end of this book.

45. Is there a way to continue my training?

Yes, all professional organisations offer further training sessions in a variety of forms.

46. When you say 'reactive reflex' what do you mean?

The client may react with verbal feed back or a physical movement. The reflexologists may recognise that the reflex feels different to what might be expected. In some cases both.

47. Can a reflexologist treat animals?

Reflexologists must not treat in the knowledge that veterinary advice has not been sought as this could lead to prosecution under the Protection of Animals Act 1911 or Veterinary Surgeons Act 1966. First aid for the purpose of saving life or relieving pain is permissible. Clear records must be kept.

48. Is there a specific reflex point for the foot?

During full treatment the foot is automatically treated. Foot reflex reactions may occur on the lateral malleous area and also on the hard heel pad in line with toes three, and four.

49. Is there a specific reflex point for the hand represented on the foot?

When giving a reflexology foot treatment the corresponding hand is benefiting. Reflex points for the hand can also be located on the lateral aspect of the foot between diaphragm and waist area. Hand reflex reactions may occur on the chest/shoulder reflex in line with toes three, four and five.

50. Do qualified reflexologists have to attend continuing professional development courses?

Yes, as part of maintaining professional memberships the therapist is expected to demonstrate evidence of attendance at a minimum of two days each year or as agreed/advised by the organisation.

REVISION QUESTIONS

1. Who brought Reflexology to America?

2. Name the American woman who specialised in Reflexology

3. How do the reflex points of Reflexology differ from the reflex points of the nervous system?

4. In Reflexology what is meant by reflex points?

5. Where are the Transverse Lines found?

6. What are the Longitudinal Zones?

7. What are the Crystals?

8. There are a number of reasons why a treatment may not be performed. List three.

9. Would you treat an Epileptic?

10. Are there any special precautions when treating a Diabetic?

11. What might happen if you over-treated a client?

12. Is it within the power of a Reflexologist to refer people to their own doctor?

13. List 4 situations when caution is required prior to, or during, treatment.

14. List seven rules of personal hygiene.

15. Name a contagious condition that affects the feet.

16. Who was Sir Henry Head?

17. What do the letters C.A.M. stand for?

18. Why is the comfort of both therapist and client important?

19. Briefly define energy.

20. While performing the initial foot examination, what is the therapist looking for or observing on the feet?

21. Why is it important for the client to see the therapist's face?

22. Why is it not advisable to use oil or cream during Reflexology treatment?

23. If a Therapist thinks it is necessary to treat with an oil, cream or talcum powder, then at what stage in the treatment might these products be used?

24. What homecare advice would you give to a client with excessively sweaty feet?

25. How much time would you allow for a first visit?

26. What sort of situation would dictate that the treatment should be given for 5/10 minutes instead of 40/45?

27. How does the treatment of a child differ from the treatment of an adult?

28. What rationale is given by some reflexologists who feel talcum powder should not be used in a Reflexology treatment?

29. What action does the therapist take when a crystal or sensitivity is felt?

30. Name the first area to be treated in the Reflexology routine.

31. In what zone does the head and brain lie?

32. Where would you treat for the pituitary gland?

33. Over what area on the foot is the spine treated?

34. In the 'Reflexology Routine' what reflex area would you be working on between Zone 1 to Zone 5 between waist and pelvic floor line?

35. According to the routine in this book, which would you treat first, the kidney or the bladder?

36. Define 'Contra Indicated'.

37. What sort of reaction might a client display during treatment?

38. Might a client suffer any reactions between visits to the therapist and if so what type of reactions might be expected?

39. Why is a consultation sheet necessary?

40. Why does the client sign the consultation sheet?

Answers to all these questions are found in the text.

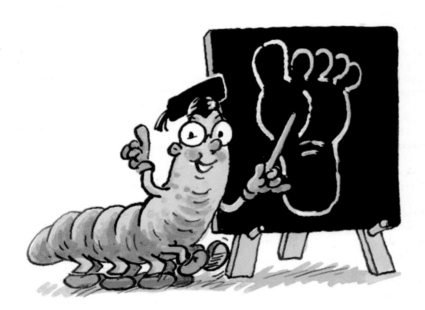

REFLEXOLOGY, ANATOMY and PHYSIOLOGY RELATED TERMS DEFINED

Abdominal
Term related to the trunk area, located below diaphragm.

Abduction
To move/take away from the mid-line, as in lifting your arm away from your body.

Adduction
Bringing towards the mid-line, as in bringing your arm close to your body.

Alternative Medicine/Therapy
Any range of therapies that fall beyond the scope of allopathic medicine but may be used alongside it to improve health and well-being. 'Alternative' is not intended to mean an alternative to allopathic medicine, it is there to offer a choice.

Anatomical Position
The body in an upright position, facing forwards, feet slightly apart, hands hanging down, palms forward.

Ankle High Spot
The prominence located on the centre of the ankle protuberance.

Artery
A thick walled blood vessel that carries oxygenated blood from the heart around the body (the aorta) and deoxygenated blood from the heart to the lungs for oxygenation (pulmonary artery).

Axillary
Term related to the armpit area.

Back up Reflex
A reflex that is treated to aid the functioning of an organ, gland or structure because it is indirectly involved in its maximum functional ability.

Ball of the Foot
The fat pad of the foot beneath the toes, corresponding to the chest area in the body. When the toes are pushed backwards the ball of the foot looks like it is sticking its chest out.

Ball/Bulb of Toe
Fat pad behind the nail on plantar of toe.

Brachial
Related to the arm area (upper limb – shoulder to elbow).

Bursa
A fluid filled pad that acts as a cushion at a pressure point in the body, often near a joint where a tendon or muscle crosses the bone or other muscles. Major bursas are at the elbow, knee and shoulder. A bursa can become inflamed, usually due to friction and this causes the condition bursitis.

Calcaneal
Area of the heel of the foot.

Carpal
Term related to the wrist area.

Case History
A record of a client's personal details taken at the first visit, examined and updated prior to any further treatment.

Caution
When a condition/disease calls for extra care or expertise on the part of the reflexologist.

Cephalic
Relates to the head area.

Cervical
Relates to a neck area.

Clinic
A place where qualified practitioners will offer a range of treatments to enhance well-being and heal ailments.

Clinical Trial
A research study in which a treatment or therapy is tested. Results of trials can also contribute to our understanding of disease and conditions, for example, how a disease progresses or how it affects different systems.

Coeliac
Relates to the area of the abdomen.

Complementary Medicine/Therapy
This 'complements' the needs of the client at physical, mental, emotional and life energy levels.

Continual Professional Development (C.P.D)
Continuing Professional Development means a progression of knowledge, a broadening of understanding. It is further study to improve on current knowledge/skill. Ongoing study.

Conventional Medicine
Medicine as practiced by a medically qualified doctor.

Costal
Related to the rib area.

Cranial
Related to the skull area.

Cubital
Relates to the area of the elbow and forearm.

Cuboid Spot
This is the soft area (indentation) located just under (heel side) the metatarsal tuberosity on the lateral edge of the foot.

Cutaneous
Relates to the skin.

Digit
The digit is referring to the finger, the thumb, or the toe.

Distal
To be distant. An organ, gland or structure farthest from source. For example, the big toe is distal to the head. The outside of the arm is distal to the mid-line.

Distal Part of the Foot
The part of the foot furthest from the body, i.e. the toes.

Dorsal or Dorsum of the Foot
The top of the foot.

Elimination Channels
The body's means of elimination of waste, i.e. colon, lungs, lymph, kidney, skin.

Endorphins
Chemical pain killers with strong analgesic action, produced naturally in the brain.

Eversion
A turning outwards, commonly applied to the foot.

Femoral
Thigh area, lower limb, hip to knee.

Forearm
Upper limb, area from elbow to wrist.

Frontal
Forehead area.

Gluteals
The buttocks

Groin
Depressed area between abdomen and thigh.

Grounding
This is sometimes practised by the therapist/practitioner prior to giving a reflexology treatment. It involves clearing the mind and invoking self protection, in that the reflexologist ensures that he/she does not psychologically take on any of the conditions which may be presented by their client. Examples of 'Grounding' can be: running cold water over the hands before and after treatment, visualising a protective barrier around you, praying, covering the solar plexus with the hands and breathing deeply and calmly. The practice of 'Grounding' can take many different forms.

Hallux
Big toe.

Healing
Our body's natural ability to repair itself. It operates at the levels of mind, body and spirit.

Helper Areas
Additional reflex areas worked to help the specific area of problem/congestion. They are areas that may have a direct or indirect effect on the reflex, e.g. a neck pain might benefit not only from the treatment on the neck but also from treatment on the cervical and thoracic spine and the shoulders.

Heredity/Hereditary
Qualities passed from parent to child.

Homeostasis
Translated from the Greek language to mean equilibrium or balance.

Holism
In 1926 Jan Christian Smuts introduced the term 'holism' as a way of viewing living things as 'entities greater than and different from the sum of their parts'.

Holistic Medicine Therapy
The art and science of healing that focuses on the whole person: body, mind and spirit. Holistic therapists encourage client education and self-help.

Inguinal
Related to the area of the groin.

Intuition
The aspect of the mental faculties which relies on non-logical modes of understanding beyond reason or physical perception.

Inversion
A turning inwards, commonly applied to the foot.

Landmarks
Physical features of the foot which can be used to orientate the reflexologist. For example, the toes, the diaphragm line.

Lateral Side of the Foot
The outside of the foot, the little toe side of the foot.

Ligament
A tough band of slightly elastic tissue that binds bone to bone at the joints, in order to prevent excessive movement. Ligaments also support the bladder, liver, uterus, diaphragm and others.

Lighter Pressure
This term indicates the use of a pressure lighter than that which would normally be considered suitable for a similar client in good health or when comparing the treatment of a child to an adult.

Lumbar region
Loin, lower back and side, rib to pelvis.

Malleolus
Malleolus *Medial* – inside ankle bone.
Malleolus *Lateral* – outside ankle bone.

Mammary
Term related to the breasts.

Medial Side of the Foot
The inside of the foot, the big toe or great toe side of the foot.

Median Line
An imaginary line, running through the centre of the body from the crown of the head to between the feet.

Metatarsal Tuberosity
The metatarsal notch is located as you run your thumb or finger down the lateral edge of the foot until you reach a bony protrusion. This is the 5th metatarsal tuberosity, sometimes easier to locate by working the hand towards the toe (from soft spot).

Metatarsal Pad
Is the ball of the foot. See Ball of Foot above.

Muscle
A structure of specialised cells capable of contraction and relaxation to create movement. There are three types of muscle: cardiac, smooth and skeletal.

Occipital
Shell shaped bone at the base of the skull, covered by muscle. The foramen magnum is a large hole in the occipital for nerve and spine inlet/outlet.

Open Questions
Questions phrased in such a way as to encourage the client to share more detail.

Opthalmic
Related to the eye area.

Oral
Related to the mouth area.

Orbital Cavity
Bony cavity, containing the eyeball.

Palmar
Term relating to the palm of the hand.

Paralanguage
Intentional contours that can be used to communicate attitudes. In the context of communication within the clinic environment it could be defined as sounds that acknowledge. For example: the question from therapist to client might be "are you warm enough?" The client's response is "Mmm…"

Paraphrasing
Repeating the main points of conversation back to the client. It allows the therapist to identify main points in the conversation (to get to the heart of the matter).

Patellar
Related to the knee.

Pectoral
Related to the area of the chest.

Pedis
Term related to the foot area.

Perineal
Area from the anus to the pubic arch.

Peripheral Neuropathy
Impairment of sensory pathway.

Personal Development
The on-going development of self-awareness, taking responsibility for own health – body, mind and spirit.

Phalange
The phalange relates to a bone in the finger or toe e.g. the distal phalange relates to the bone nearest to the top of the finger or toe (the first joint that includes the nail).

Placebo
A result due to a patient's/client's belief in that treatment.

Plantar Surface of the Foot
The sole or bottom of the foot.

Pollex
This is the thumb.

Popliteal
The area behind the knee.

Proximal
An organ or structure closest to the source. For example, the inside of the arm is proximal to the mid-line.

Proximal Part of the Foot
The part of the foot nearest to the body i.e. the heel is proximal to the head. The toe is distal to the head.

Sacral area
Around the base of the spine.

Solar Plexus, Coeliac Plexus
The solar plexus is commonly referred to as the abdominal brain. It channels information between the brain and the nerves to all organs in the abdomen, regulating many functions and triggering when necessary emergency responses such as conveying fight or flight instructions from the brain to the adrenal glands. Amongst its many duties the solar plexus sends reminders to the stomach to digest food, the kidney to eliminate waste and the liver to produce bile. Treatment at the beginning and end of a reflexology sequence is a must in the maintenance of good health and best practice.

Tarsals
Ankle bones.

Tendon
Strong, flexible inelastic fibrous cord that binds muscle to muscle or muscle to bone.

Thenar Eminence
Heel of hand, i.e. the fat pad on the palm, under the thumb.

Thoracic region
The chest, trunk between neck and diaphragm.

Vein
A blood vessel that carries de-oxygenated blood from the capillaries back to the heart (from the rest of the body). Pulmonary veins carry oxygenated blood to the heart. Veins have valves to prevent back flow. Weak valves are responsible for varicose veins.

Umbilical
Naval area, site of umbilical cord entry.

Zones
The ten imaginary channels or zones dividing the body longitudinally from head to foot. Five zones divide each foot and hand in a similar way.

ANATOMICAL DESCRIPTIONS OF LOCATIONS

Term	Meaning/Location	Term	Meaning/Location
Superior	Toward the head/upper part	Visceral	Pertaining to an internal organ
Inferior (caudad)	Toward the feet/lower part	Ipsilateral	On the same side of the body
Anterior (ventral)	Front surface	Contralateral	On the opposite side of the body
Posterior (dorsal)	Rear surface	**Body Planes**	
Superficial	Toward the surface of the body	Sagittal	Divides into right and left
Deep	Away from the body surface	Transverse	Divides superior and inferior
Parietal	Forming wall of body cavity	Frontal (coronal)	Divides anterior and posterior

USEFUL INFORMATION

If You Are An Apprehensive Prospective Client: What can you expect from a Reflexology treatment?

A client should expect an introductory chat with the Reflexologist before they begin treatment. This should include the completion of a consultation sheet – (See page 114) Once formal consent has been given, following signatures from the client and the Reflexologist, treatment can commence, providing no contra indications have been identified (See pages 61 - 75).

The Reflexologist will begin work on the feet, or hands, if appropriate, and will take note (usually mentally) of any problem areas. Clients may experience some discomfort in certain areas, however this will usually be brief, this may indicate areas of imbalance in the body. Generally the treatment will feel wonderful, relaxing and soothing.

The first treatment (including the chat and completion of the consultation sheet) will take around an hour and 15 minutes. The subsequent treatments will generally last around 45 minutes. A course of treatments can vary depending on individual needs and can be discussed with the Reflexologist.

How will I feel?
A client will generally feel well and relaxed after treatment however everyone's body is different and can respond in individual ways. Possible side effects can be discussed with the Reflexologist and symptoms can vary widely. Do not be alarmed or worried by any slight side effects, these are usually a reflection that the treatment is working and your body is responding in a positive way.

Always check that your practitioner/therapist is a qualified Reflexologist and a member of a recognised Reflexology organisation.

There are 3 Treatment Types:

3 types of reflexology treatment are commonly referred to:

i)   **Causal**
ii)   **Symptomatic**
iii)   **Urgent Care Routine**

i)   **Causal Treatment**
     The type generally given by a professional therapist. All reflexes are treated and further treatment given to specific reflexes as appropriate.

ii) **Symptomatic Treatment**
     Symptomatic treatment as the name suggests deals with the reflexes related to the symptom and may also employ some support reflexes, i.e. neck ache could have support reflex of shoulder treated.

iii) **Urgent Care Routine**
     Devised by myself many years ago and used when a specific gentle treatment is given to clear energy pathways, improve breathing and bring about general relaxation. (See Page 92)

STUDENT SUPPORT INFORMATION

Complementary Therapies

In all my years of teaching I guided students and encouraged them to guide others to study and have a basic understanding of the complementary therapies that are widely available. To aid study, I suggest a medium sized (A5) index card be used to record a basic definition of the therapy, what is involved in the treatment and the most common uses and suitability of the treatment alongside, or as an alternative to, reflexology. This knowledge will be valuable in ensuring best practice and for referral purposes.

To have an understanding of other complementary disciplines therapists should be aware of the following facts:

- What does it involve?
- What type of treatment is it?
- Can one receive it alongside Reflexology?

List of Disciplines

Acupressure, Acupuncture, Alexander Technique, Aromatherapy, Bach Flower Remedies, Bowen Technique, Chiropractic, Healing – spiritual and natural, Herbalism, Homeopathy, Hypnotherapy, Iridology, Kinesiology, Neurolinguistic Programming (NLP), Osteopathy, Physiotherapy, Reiki, Remedial and Therapeutic Massage, Shiatsu, Therapeutic Touch, Traditional Chinese Medicine, Yoga.

Therapists should know which of the above therapies would be most suited for specific conditions, for example, structural problems would be best suited to the Alexander Technique, Chiropractic and Osteopathy. Systemic conditions, such as eczema would be suited to Herbal Medicine, Homeopathy and T.C.M (Traditional Chinese Medicine). Therapists should understand epilation (Electrolysis). This is a treatment commonly used in the treatment of hair growth problems, associated with endocrine disorders in females.

General Therapies

Electrolysis

The common name used for methods of permanent removal of unwanted hair. A needle is passed into the hair follicle and a current of electricity is discharged to destroy the germinating cells either by chemical galvanic means or by short wave diathermy. Clients presenting with endocrine disorders may be undergoing treatment with electrolysis as abnormal hair growth may a side effect of the disorder.

Podiatry – Chiropody – Pedicure
As all these disciplines are involved in the maintenance of healthy feet an awareness
of each modality will be of value to both client and therapist.

Disorders, Diseases, Conditions
In line with my teachings over the years I advise all those interested in Reflexology to
make their own reference file. This can be achieved manually with a ready-reference
index card and box system or on the computer.

Initially the reference should be established with a list of 25 of the most common
disorders. This list can be expanded with time.

Suggested Layout:

- Basic definition of condition
- Usual symptoms and medical treatment
- A list of reflexes and support reflexes to assist healing.
- Rationale

Medical Specialists
A knowledge and understanding of the role of the medical specialist will support the
therapist in an aim to give holistic care. The knowledge for the client can be the key to
further investigation and understanding. Examples of these are: cardiologist,
endocrinologist, dermatologist, gynaecologist, haematologist, oncologist,
opthamologist, orthopaedic specialist, pathologist, paediatrician, proctologist,
rheumatologist.

Student Record Keeping
All written records on clients used for course work or case studies should have any
sensitive information or personal details removed before the work is seen by another
person. Clients can be identified or indexed by using either colour or numeric coding.
The student can keep a secure master/key file away from the portfolio. For verification
purposes client's details may be requested by a tutor or external examiner. Agreement
should be obtained from the client for such information to be given to a third party.

THERAPIST AND STUDENT SUPPORT INFORMATION

Data Protection
All recorded information, both written and electronic, must conform to the Data Protection Act.

Interpersonal Distance
The following is a guide to the divisions of interpersonal distance in relation to the practice of reflexology:

Intimate space: 0" – 18"   (0cm - 45cm) lovers and intimate family
Personal space: 4" – 18"   (10cm - 45cm) friends
Social space: 4" – 12"   (10cm - 30cm) business and casual acquaintances
Public space: 12" – 25"   (30cm - 63cm) formal interactions

Preparing Self
The therapist should maintain their own health through good diet and lifestyle. Avoid becoming exhausted by treating only an appropriate number of clients in a working day and by taking breaks between treatments.

Support Services – Voluntary and Statutory Organisations
All practitioners should appreciate that voluntary and statutory support services may have a role in managing a client's condition. It may help the client if the practitioner is aware of the support services available in order to make recommendations to the client, where appropriate.

Voluntary
The practitioner should be aware of the focus areas and the range of organisations available to offer support and advice. For example, Cruse, WRVS, Age Concern, Help the Aged, RNIB, RNID, CAB, Samaritans, RELATE, AA, AIDS Helpline.

Statutory
Examples are, the Social Services, the Benefits Agency, Local Borough Housing Departments, Medical or Health Centres, NHS Advice Line/Alert.

CURRENT LEGISLATION

- Cancer Act 1939
- Care Standards Act 2000
- Children Act 1989
- Children (leaving care) Act 2000
- Control of Diseases Act 1984
- Control of Diseases Regulations Act 1988
- Control of Substances Hazardous to Health Regulations (COSHH) 1999
- Crime and Disorder Act 1998
- Dangerous Substances and Preparations (nickel) 2000
- Data Protection Act 1984
- Disability Discrimination Act 1995
- Electricity at Work 1989
- Employers Liability Act 1969
- Environmental Protection Act 1990
- ECHR (Human Rights Act) 1998
- Fire Precautions Act 1971
- Fire Precautions (Workplace) Regulations 1997
- Health and Safety (First Aid) Act 1981
- Health and Safety at Work Act 1974
- Local Government (Miscellaneous Provisions) Act 1982
- Management of Health and Safety at Work 1999
- Medical Act 1983
- Performing Rights (under Copyright Designs and Patents) Act 1988
- Personal Protective Equipment Act 1992
- Protection of Children Act 1999
- Provision and Use of Work Equipment 1992
- Race Relations Act 1976
- Reporting Injuries, Diseases and Dangerous Occurrences (RIDDOR) 1995
- Sale and Supply of Goods Act 1994
- Sex Discrimination Act 1986

- Sex Offenders Act 1997
- Social Services Act 1970 (Section 7)
- Trades Description Act 1972
- VAT Act 1994
- Venereal Disease Act 1917
- Work Place Regulations (Health, Safety and Welfare) 1992
- Working Time Regulations 1998
- Youth Justice and Criminal Evidence Act 1999

Reflexologists should also be aware of:

- Codes of Ethics and Practice of any professional body which the reflexologist may intend to join.
- Local Authority Licensing Regulations
- Local Authority planning requirements for clinics and working from home
- Local Environmental Health Regulations
- Recognised Industry Codes of Ethics and Practice

Note

The G.M.C.'s rules for doctors, published in 'Professional Conduct and Discipline Fitness to Practice', dated February 1991 (paragraph 42 and 43) allow a doctor to delegate to persons trained to perform special functions, treatment or procedures, provided that the doctor retains ultimate responsibility for the management of the patient.

The UK Government statement of December 3rd 1991 confirmed the doctor's right to delegate treatment of patients to specialists, including complementary therapists.

Such treatment can be paid for by either the health authority or by the GP's practice.

THE LAW

UK law is enshrined in a series of Acts and Statutes principally associated with the medical and paramedical professions. It is the responsibility of the reflexologist to ensure that he/she is not breaking the law of the country in which they are working

Reflexologists should know it is an offence to advertise in a way that would imply that they treat a variety of conditions including those listed here

In the United Kingdom it is an offence for Reflexologists to advertise that they treat the following: Bright's Disease (nephritis), Cancer, Cataracts, Diabetes, Epilepsy, Glaucoma, Locomotor Ataxy, Paralysis, Tuberculosis or Venereal Disease.

It is not an offence to offer a reflexology treatment in support of medical treatment
- reflexologists must not treat a client in any case which exceeds their capability, training and competence. Where appropriate, the reflexologist must seek referral to a suitably qualified person,
- reflexologists must never make a medical diagnosis or countermand the advice of a medical doctor',
- reflexologists must not treat a young person under the age of 18 years without first obtaining the written consent of the parent or guardian,
- The parent or guardian should be present during the treatment of a young person under the age of 16 years
- The parent or guardian withholding medical care from a minor/ young person could be committing a criminal offence
- reflexologists who become aware that the client is suffering with a notifiable or infectious disease must advise the client to seek urgent medical help and to avoid contact with others. In extreme cases it may become necessary that the reflexologist contacts the client's GP or Public Health department.

UK CHARITIES
SOME USEFUL
NAMES AND NUMBERS

This list is not exhaustive

NAME	CONTACT
Allergy UK	020 8303 8525
Alzheimer's Research Trust	www.alzheimers-research.org.uk 01223 843899
Arthritis Research Campaign	www.arc.org.uk 01246 558033
Blood Pressure Association	www.bpassoc.org.uk 020 8772 4985
Brain and Spine Foundation	www.brainandspine.org.uk 020 7793 5900
British Council for Disabled People	01332 295551
British Heart Foundation	020 7935 0185
British Vascular Foundation	www.bvf.org.uk 01483 726511
Cancer Research UK	www.cancerresearchuk.org 020 7009 8833
Colon and Rectal Disease Research Foundation of GB and Ireland	01244 365445
Community Health UK	01273 234868
Diabetes UK	020 7424 1000
Down's Syndrome Association	www.downs-syndrome.org.uk 020 8682 4001
Drug Scope	020 7928 1211
Drugs Prevention Advisory Service	www.homeoffice.gov.uk/takingdrugs 0800 776 600

NAME	CONTACT
Eating Disorders Association	0845 634 1414 Helpline
Epilepsy Action	0113 210 8800
Epilepsy: The Fund for Epilepsy	01422 823508
European Association for the Treatment of Addiction (UK)	www.eata.org.uk 020 7922 8753
Institution of Occupational Safety and Health	0116 257 3100
International Glaucoma Association	020 7737 3265
Leonard Cheshire Foundation	020 7802 8200
Marie Curie Cancer Care	0800 716146
Meningitis Research Foundation	01454 281811
Migraine Trust	020 7831 4818
MIND	www.mind.org.uk 020 8215 2243
Multiple Sclerosis Society	020 8438 0700
National Association for Colitis and Crohn's Disease (NACC)	01727 830038
National Autistic Society	020 7833 2299
National Benevolent Fund for the Aged	020 8688 6655
National Eczema Society	020 7281 3553

NAME	CONTACT
National Kidney Research Fund	01733 704656
National Society for the Prevention of Cruelty to Children (NSPCC)	020 7825 2500
Neuro-Disability Research Trust	020 8780 4568
No Panic (Support for Sufferers of Anxiety Disorder)	01952 590005
Obesity Awareness and Solutions Trust	01279 866010
Pain Relief Foundation	www.painrelieffoundation.org.uk 0151 529 5820
Prostate Cancer Charity	020 8222 7622
Psoriasis Association	01604 711129
QUIT (Support for Smokers to give up)	0800 002200
Repetitive Strain Injury Association	020 7266 2000
Roy Castle Lung Cancer Foundation	0871 220 5426
Royal National Institute for Deaf People (RNID)	0141 554 0053
Royal National Institute of the Blind (RNIB)	www.rnib.org.uk 020 8438 9076
Royal Society for the Prevention of Accidents	0121 248 2000
Royal Society for the Promotion of Health	020 7630 0121
Skin Treatment and Research Trust (START)	020 8746 8174

NAME	CONTACT
St Dunstan's (for blind ex-Service men and women)	www.st-dunstans.org.uk 020 7723 5021
Stroke Association	www.stroke.org.uk 020 7566 0300
Terrence Higgins Trust (AIDS & HIV)	www.tht.org.uk 0845 122 1200
WellBeing, the Health Research Charity for Women and Babies	020 7772 6400
WellWomen Information	0117 941 2983
World Cancer Research Fund	www.wcrf-uk.org 020 7343 4200

FINALLY

No person or book can teach you what you will gain from experience and consolidation. A minimum of one year should be given over to laying the foundations after you qualify. The professional must continue to update knowledge and never become complacent.

My mission is through reflexology and continued new knowledge of the subject to work towards better health for everyone.

Enjoy Reflexology!

Renée.

ORGANISATION ADDRESSES

Australia
Reflexology Association of Australia
PO Box 366, Cammeray, NSW 2062, Australia
Tel: 61 02 4721 4752 Fax: 61 02 9631 3287

Austria
Academy of Reflexology Austria
Achsengraben 12, A-4230 Pregarten

Belgium
Centre d'Etude de Reflexologie
Avenue H. et F. Limbourg, 29 bte 3, 1070 Bruxelles, Belgium
Tel et Fax: 32 2 524 25 64 Email: yves.vanopdenbosch@village.uunet.be

Canada
Reflexology Association of Canada (RAC)
#201, 17930-105 Avenue, Edmonton, Alberta T5S 2H5, Canada
Tel: 1 780 443 4246 Fax: 1 780 444 6882

China
Chinese Society of Reflexologists
Xuanwu Hospital, Capital Institute of Medicine, Chang Chun Street,
Beijing, China

Denmark
Forenede Danske Zoneterapeuter (Danish Reflexologists Association)
Secretariat, Overgade 14, 1.tv. 5000 Odense, Denmark
Tel: 45 70 278850 Fax: 45 70 279950 Email: info@fdz.dk

Finland
Association of Finnish Reflexologists
Albertinkatu 5, 00150 Helsinki, Finland
Tel: 358 50 5227766 Fax: 358 9 6225160

France
Federation Francais des Reflexologues
60 Rue de la Colonie, 75013 Paris, France
Tel: 33 14 534 2403 Email: pviricel@wanadoo.fr

Germany
Deutscher Reflexologen Verband (DRV)
Hakenfelder Str. 9A, D-13587 Berlin, Germany
Tel & Fax: 49 30 337 93 16

Greece
Hellenic Association of Reflexologists
84 Alkionis Str, P. Faliro 17562, Athens, Greece

India
Indian Society for Promotion of Reflexology
D-6-B M.I.G. Flats, G-8 Area (Rajouri Garden), Mayapuri,
New Delhi-110064, India
Tel/Fax: 91 11 3711018 or 91 11 5490005 Email: gfchowallur@yahoo.co.in

Ireland
National Register of Reflexologists (Ireland)
The Registrar, Unit 13, Upper Mall, Terryland Retail Park, Headford Road,
Galway, Ireland
Tel: 353 91 568844

Israel
Israeli Reflexology Association
PO Box 39220, Tel Aviv 61391, Israel
Italy
Federatzione Italiana di Reflessologia del Piede
c/o MEDIA - Piazza Locatelli 10, 24043 CARAVAGGIO BG, Italy
Tel: 39 0363 350135 Fax: 39 0363 350654

Japan
Japan Reflexologist Education College
Refle Building, 2-22-23 Higashi-Nakano, Nakano-Ku,
Tokyo 164-0003, Japan
Tel: 0120-708-531 03-3367-8531 Email: info@refle.co.jp

Netherlands
Vereniging Van Nederlands Reflexzone Therapeuten
't Prooyen 5, 1141 VD Monnickendam, Netherlands
Tel: 31 299 652882 Fax: 31 299 655240

New Zealand
New Zealand Reflexology Association
PO Box 31 084, Auckland 9, New Zealand
Tel: 64 9 486 1918 Fax: 64 9 489 2916

Norway
Norsk Forening For Soneterapeuter
Sverresgate 33, 5100 Bergen, Norway
Tel: 47 5523 0430 Fax: 47 5593 1644

Poland
Polish Instytut of Reflexology
20-553 Lublin ul.Hetmanska 8/2
Tel: 48 81 442 82 82 Fax: 1 905 227 5997
Email: awbratko@warplink.com

Portugal
Association of Reflexology (AR) Portugal
Rua de Santa Catarina, 722 - 3dto, 4000 Oporto, Portugal
Email: arportugal@mail.telepac.pt

South Africa
The South African Reflexology Society
PO Box 18850, Dalbridge, 4014, South Africa
Tel/Fax: 27 31 2054518 Email: admin@sareflexology.org.za

Sweden
Svenska Fotzonterapeuters Rikforbund
Alvdansvagen 15, 436 42 Askim, Sweden
Tel: 46 31 280230 Fax: 46 31 286160

Switzerland
Association Suisse D'Etude de la Reflexologie
2001 Neuchatel, Casa Postale 126, Switzerland
Tel: 41 38 41 29 21 Fax: 41 38 41 28 20

United Kingdom
Association of Reflexologists
27 Old Gloucester Street, London WC1N 3XX, England
Tel: 44 870 5673320 Fax: 44 1823 336646 Email: Info@aor.org

British Reflexology Association
Monks Orchard, Whitbourne, Worcester WR6 5RB, England
Tel: 44 1886 821207 Fax: 44 1886 822017 Email: Bra@britreflex.co.uk

International Federation of Reflexologists
76-78 Edridge Road, Croydon, Surrey CR0 1EF, England
Tel: 44 208 645 9134 Fax: 44 208 649 9192
Email: info@IntFedReflexologists.org

International Guild of Professional Practitioners
4 Heathfield Terrace, Chiswick, London, W4 4JE, England
Tel: 44 020 8994 7856 Fax: 44 020 8994 7880 Email: guild@igpp.co.uk

International Institute of Reflexology (UK)
146 Upperthorpe, Walkley, Sheffield, S6 3NF, England
Tel/Fax: 44 1142 812100 Email: info@reflexology-uk.net

Professional Association of Clinical Therapists
3rd Floor, Eastleigh House, Upper Market Street,
Eastleigh, Hampshire, SO50 9FD, England
Tel: 44 870 420 20 22 Fax: 44 23 8048 8970 Email: info@fht.org.uk

Reflexologists Society
39 Prestbury Road, Cheltenham, Gloucestershire GL52 2PT, England
Tel: 44 1242 512601

Reflexology Practitioners Association
PO Box 36248, London SE19 3YD, England
Tel/Fax: 44 208 680 7761

Scottish Institute of Reflexology
4 Eden Road, Ednam, Kelso TD5 7QG, Scotland
Tel: 44 141 773 0018 Email: info@Scottishreflexology.org

United States of America
Foot Reflex Awareness Association
PO Box 7622, Mission Hills, California 91346, USA

Professional Association of Reflexologists of New Mexico
PO Box 27292, Albuquerque, New Mexico 87125-7292, USA

INDEX

Index

287

V

W

Y

Z

SUPPORT MATERIALS

FULL COLOUR REFLEXOLOGY CHART

STEP BY STEP REFLEXOLOGY VIDEO

STEP BY STEP REFLEXOLOGY DVD

OTHER BOOKS BY Renée Tanner

FOOTREADING

REFLEXOLOGY THE CASE HISTORY BOOK

REFLEXOLOGY THE QUESTION & ANSWER BOOK

STEP BY STEP AROMATHERAPY